HERBS
AND MEDICINAL PLANTS

MADGE HOOPER

Illustrated by
Sarah De Ath
and George Thompson

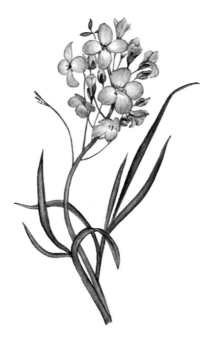

Kingfisher Books

First published in 1984 by Kingfisher Books Limited
Elsley Court, 20–22 Great Titchfield Street
London W1P 7AD
A Grisewood & Dempsey Company

BRITISH LIBRARY CATALOGUING IN PUBLICATION DATA
Hooper, Madge
   Kingfisher guide to herbs and medicinal
   plants. – (Kingfisher guides)
   1. Herbs   2. Medicinal plants
   I. Title
   641.3'57   SB351.H5
   ISBN 0 86272 094 X

Edited by Caroline Royds
Black and white illustrations by Sheila Hadley
References for illustrations by Jill Foster
Colour separations by Newsele Litho, Milan, London
Phototypeset by Southern Positives and Negatives (SPAN),
Lingfield, Surrey
Printed and bound in Italy by Vallardi Industrie
Grafiche, Milan

CONTENTS

Introduction	9
Herb Families	20
Poisonous Herbs	117
Glossary	122
Index	123

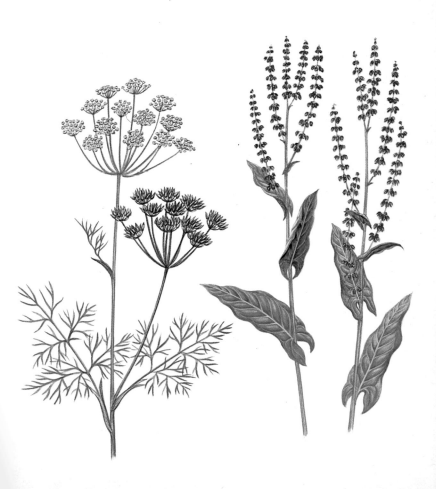

Aneti..

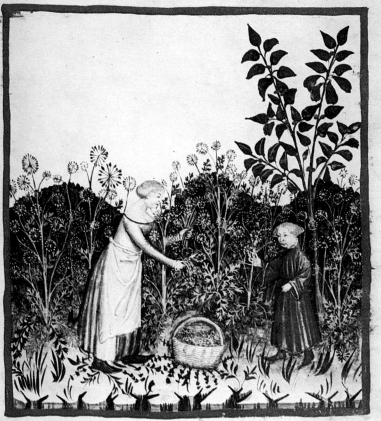

Aneti. ⟨pplo⟩. cꝰa.ſic.inſine. ſi.uſ pancipio.etꝰ .Acerõ uirtꝰ recens ⁊ tenꝟum. uniamꝰum. oſer
ſtõ ſto⁊ uentoſo. noꝛumanm noꝛt renib⟨ abominat ſcõm ſua ſba. Remõ noꝛuman eulæn
cellis. Qnõ gnꝝꝝ nutrumentũ malicũ, oſert ſtõꝝ huis ſcibꝝ. hyemeꝛ ſtꝝ regionibꝝ.

al ouenmꝰ

INTRODUCTION

Over thousands of years, herbs have been used as food, or to make food more palatable, as important drugs and simple medicinal remedies, and as sweet-smelling plants which give pleasure. The earliest cave-dwellers discovered that eating certain plants improved their diet and health. They also found that plants could provide fibre for clothing and dyes to colour body and fabric, and could be used to make signs, drawings and paintings. Most important of all, perhaps, certain herbs could be used to relieve and sometimes cure the ailments which were an inevitable part of hard and dangerous lives.

As they moved over the earth, our ancestors found and experimented with different plants, gaining knowledge but doubtless also suffering casualties as trial and error taught which herbs were poisonous and which safe. When it was discovered that such valuable sources of food and medicine could be cultivated, people ceased to be nomads – settlements grew up and barter and trade took place between them. Travellers brought back plants and seeds, the latter sometimes accidentally attached to their clothing, which became the beginnings of flourishing new plant colonies.

Our knowledge of the history of herbs comes from a wide range of literary records from across the world. In the Bible there is a graphic account of the furnishing of the Tabernacle 'with ten curtains . . . made of fine twined linen and blue and purple and scarlet stuff'. The linen was woven from flax and the dyes almost certainly came from plants. The manna that falls like rain on the hungry fleeing Israelites is likened to coriander seed and in the New Testament mention is made of the payment of tithes of mint, rue and anise. The names mugwort and lungwort bear witness to the use of herbs in Anglo-Saxon times – 'wort' being the Anglo-Saxon word for plant or herb.

The Romans, who relished luxury and good living, used herbs in cooking and to perfume rooms and baths. When they occupied Britain, they brought herbs with them – flavours and fragrances to remind them of their warmer, sunnier homeland. In medieval times, the monks cultivated medicinal herbs in their enclosed gardens and produced careful copies of the early herbals, and in the 16th and 17th centuries, two great herbalists, Gerard and Culpeper, wrote notable treatises on the medicinal powers of herbs. Year after year, in the stillrooms of country houses, women have evolved, collected and handed down recipes (receipts) for medicines, cosmetics and conserves, and in many cases have been responsible for the health of the whole household. Fear, superstition and magic were often entangled with herbal treatment in the past but modern research, which can analyse the plants into their constituents, has finally established the sound scientific basis of much herbal medicine.

Sharing the pleasure of gathering dill in medieval times.

Growing Herbs

Herbs fit into most garden schemes, and the variety of their foliage, colours, textures, shapes and evocative scents gives constant pleasure. They will grow successfully in pots or other containers and in pockets of soil between paving stones. Favourite herbs planted in a patch of gravel make an attractive alternative to grass, with the added advantage of eliminating the need for mowing. Formally designed herb gardens and copies of the old knot gardens are delightful to look at, but need a great deal of attention to keep them in the immaculate condition they demand. Most herbs are hardy and easy to grow, but it may help to remember that many of the small-leaved aromatic plants, like thyme, rosemary and lavender, came from sunny Mediterranean countries, so they thrive best in an open, well-drained, sunny place in the garden, protected from cold east winds. Plants with big leaves, like comfrey and angelica, should be planted where the soil is rich in humus or naturally damp to provide the moisture needed for abundant leaf growth. Peat, while not providing nourishment, helps to hold moisture in a light soil and opens, aerates and assists root growth in a heavy soil. Herbs do not flourish in too rich a soil, which encourages sappy growth and deficiencies in stamina, flavour and fragrance. A dressing of manure every three years, and the using of compost at planting time, as a top dressing in autumn, and to mulch before the summer sun dries out the soil, will keep the plants growing healthily.

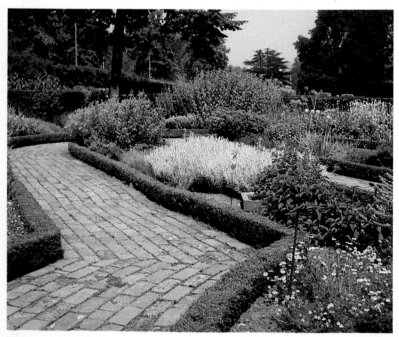

Growing from seed

Annual, biennial and perennial plants can be raised economically from seed. Spring sowing out of doors should not be done until the cold winds are over, the soil is warming up and the sun strong enough and the days long enough to encourage young seedlings to grow into healthy plants. If they are sown too early they may germinate in a short warm spell and will not maintain growth when the cold winds return. Seedlings raised under glass should not be sown so early that they need planting out before the weather is right for them. April for indoor and May for outdoor sowing is not too late. Light soils will encourage the growth of many self-sown seedlings, and recording when they emerge can be a good guide to when it is wise to start sowing.

Most of the hardy herbs will grow from seeds sown in spring but in some cases it is best to sow immediately after the seeds have ripened and some need to stratify, that is to lie out in the cold soil of winter. Each year, seed may be saved from healthy plants. In some cases, they will provide the part of the plant most used in culinary or medicinal preparations (e.g. anise, caraway and sunflower). The length of time seeds remain viable varies a good deal. Sow trial samples to test seeds that are over a year old.

The well-balanced, established herbs of a garden in Kent, combining flower and foliage colours with neatly trimmed formal edging plants and the warmth of old brick paths running between the beds.

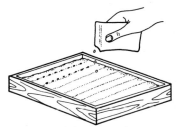

Sowing seeds in prepared compost. Big seeds may be allowed space, to eliminate pricking out.

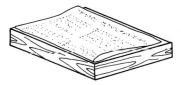

Cover box with a sheet of glass and paper to exclude light.

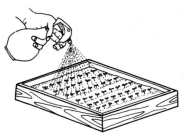

Prick out small seedlings and water with fine spray. Compost should be damp, not wet.

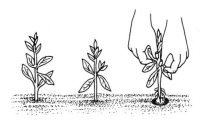

When big enough to handle, carefully plant out young seedlings to herb beds, and water if necessary.

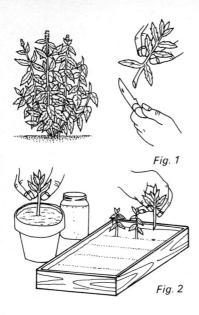

Fig. 1

Fig. 2

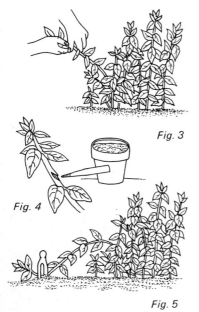

Fig. 3

Fig. 4

Fig. 5

Seed Collecting

When fully ripe, seeds will drop easily from the plant, but wait for a dry day before collecting them. Take a large enough piece of material and place it under the plants. Cut the stalks so that any seeds dropping fall on the cloth. Rub the seeds off the stalks and leave them spread out to ensure they are perfectly dry before storing them in a cool place. Plants grown from seed may sometimes be variable, showing differences in colour, leaf form and size, but those grown by vegetative propagation – by stem or root cuttings, or by layering or division of the plant – will produce young plants which come true in all characteristics to the parent plant.

Taking Cuttings

All the bushy herbs can be increased from cuttings taken in late spring or early autumn or when the atmosphere is warm and humid. The plant from which the cuttings are to be taken should be healthy. Pull off short shoots (5–8cm long) by holding the shoot near its joint with the stem and gently but firmly pulling downwards so that it comes off with a 'heel'. Or choose a healthy young shoot and cut it off, with a sharp knife or pair of secateurs, just below a node (fig. 1). Take off all leaves except a small terminal group, again pulling downwards. Then let the severed end dry a little or dip it in a hormone rooting powder. Prepare pots (clay pots are best) or boxes by spreading broken crocks or coarse clean gravel at the bottom for drainage, then fill with coarse sandy compost. Insert the cuttings into the compost (fig. 2), making them firm with your fingers. Water and put in a shady, well-ventilated place. Cuttings of most hardy herbs will root well out of doors in a semi-shady bed of soil. If the soil is heavy, sand, peat, shale, grit or compost can be added. The cuttings seem to do well set closely together. Small batches can be planted in a circle and covered by a plastic bucket set upside-down over them. If the bucket is lifted for a short while every other day or so to ventilate, this homely propagator will speed rooting.

Layering
Layering is a method of propagation by which a branch is pegged down and roots form at the point in contact with the soil. The branch is bent over (fig. 3) and will root more quicky if the underside of the stem is scraped at the node and dusted with hormone rooting powder (fig. 4). A mixture of sand and peat is scattered where it is to be pegged down into the soil (fig. 5). The potential new plant is maintained by the parent while it makes roots and it can then be detached and planted where needed.

Division
Chives, marjoram, winter savory and thyme are all plants which may be trimmed of old growth and pulled apart into smaller rooted clumps for replanting. Lovage and elecampane can be increased by digging up mature roots in spring and cutting off the pieces of root with a bud or 'eye' attached. If planted in good soil young roots will soon develop.

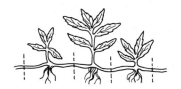

Young plants can be detached from rhizomes of mints, where they have rooted at the nodes.

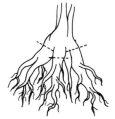

Pieces of the thick rootstock of comfrey can be cut off and replanted to make new plants.

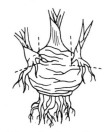

The 'buds' or shoots on the crown of elecampane or lovage roots, cut off with some root attached, form new plants.

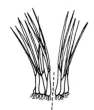

Chives and other bulbous plants can be divided into small new clumps for replanting.

Harvesting and Drying Herbs

Even a small herb garden, once it is established, can produce more growth during the summer than will be needed for immediate use, so the surplus can be dried or frozen. In drying, herbs should lose nothing but their moisture, retaining both colour and fragrance. Whether they are to be used for cooking, herb teas or in pot pourri, the principles of drying are the same. When the herb is coming into flower, the oil content of the plant and the source of flavour and scent held in the stem and leaves are at their highest, so when possible this is the best time to harvest them.

To dry herbs well they need a steady circulation of heat, and light must be excluded to preserve their colour. Trying to dry them by hanging them in bunches in an airy place will usually lead to disappointment. The inside of a bunch does not dry as quickly as the outside, and the airy place may be dry during the day and moist at night. On a commercial scale, the best quality herbs are spread on racks in a darkened shed with artificial heat maintained at something over 27°C (80°F). At home, the airing cupboard with its slatted shelves over the hot water cylinder makes an ideal place to dry small quantities of herbs and flowers. Some very loosely woven material or netting can be spread over the shelves, the herbs can be put in baskets or, best of all, in one or two wooden or metal framed sieves, diameter 35cm or 45cm with mesh 0.6cm ($\frac{1}{4}$in.) and 0.3cm ($\frac{1}{8}$in.).

The herbs should be cut on a dry morning when the dew is gone, and

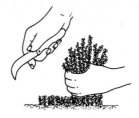

1. Cut herbs a little above ground level to avoid leaves mud-splashed from rain.

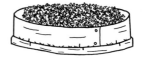

2. Fill the sieve with lightly packed cut herbs.

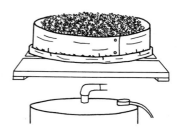

3. Place sieve in a warm airing cupboard or other warm, darkish place, to dry.

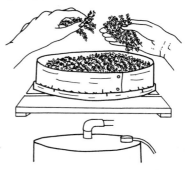

4. Lightly turn herbs daily to ensure even drying. Do not bruise leaves when handling them.

before the sun gets too hot. Always cut the plants a few centimetres above ground level to avoid any mud-splashed leaves, and discard those which are discoloured. Fresh herbs should be handled as little as possible to avoid bruising them – once they have lost their colour they cannot regain it. Put the herbs into the sieves and then the sieves into the airing cupboard. Turn the herbs over carefully the following day and each day after that till they are crisp and the stems snap when bent; 3–5 days is usually long enough for them to dry, but small-leaved herbs like thyme dry more quickly than those with bigger, fleshier leaves.

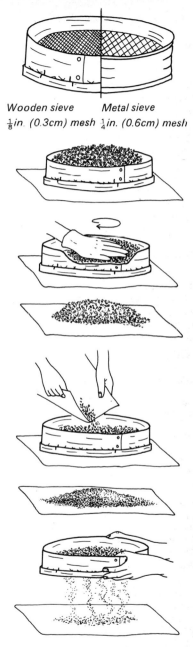

Wooden sieve   Metal sieve
$\frac{1}{8}$in. (0.3cm) mesh $\frac{1}{4}$in. (0.6cm) mesh

Preparing Dried Herbs

When all the material is completely dry, take the sieve from the airing cupboard and put some sheets of clean paper on a table. Wearing a glove to avoid getting splinters in the palm, rub the herbs through the mesh with a firm circular move-ment of the flat hand so that the stalks lie horizontally on top of the sieve and the crushed herb falls through. Throw away the big stalks, tip the rubbed herbs back into the sieve and repeat the process.

If the herb is to be used as an infusion, two rubs through the $\frac{1}{4}$in. mesh will be sufficient to get rid of most of the stalks. Herbs to be used in cooking should be rubbed through the $\frac{1}{8}$in. mesh, reducing the size of the rubbed herb and eliminating all stalks. A close mesh metal, hair or nylon sieve is useful to shake the rubbed herbs in: any dust will fall through, leaving the herbs clean and ready for storing.

15

Storing Herbs

It is as important to store herbs out of direct light as it is to dry them in the dark. They should be kept in glass jars with well-fitting screw on lids lined with greaseproof paper or foil. For large quantities, use strong brown paper bags enclosed in plastic bags and carefully sealed with twist ties. With the exception of parsley, which always fades after a few months, herbs stored in these conditions should last until the following summer's crops can replace them.

Herbs for freezing should be carefully selected, washed and shaken free of excess moisture. They can then be packed in the small amounts usually needed, and stored together in clearly labelled bags or boxes. Parsley, thyme, sage, rosemary and bay usually survive the winter and can be picked fresh from the garden, but well dried herbs make welcome presents for friends without gardens. Bay leaves should be picked when they are quite dry, and only the stiff, mature leaves used. If they are loosely wrapped, ten at a time, in greaseproof paper or foil, and then enclosed in sealed brown paper bags, they will stay a good green colour for some time. Dried bay leaves will lose their colour and break up. The subtle use of herbs in cooking is an old skill which is being relearned in this country, and one which offers endless opportunities to explore the scope of a wide variety of herbs. The best cooks are not always the ones who use the same recipes every time, but those with the flair to experiment.

Making Pot Pourri

The flowers and scented herbs used in pot pourri dry excellently in the airing cupboard. Rose petals, the most important ingredient, should be taken from fully open roses the day before they would have dropped (this soon becomes easy to judge). Cornflowers, marigolds and delphiniums have no scent but they add good colour to the mixture. Some flowers, particularly those which grow from spring bulbs, do not hold their colour well, but it is best to experiment at first with what is in your garden. Lavender, rosemary, scented mints, clove carnations, lemon verbena, bergamot and other scented flowers, blended with rose petals, will make a delightful pot pourri. It is tempting to try out the recipes in old herb books, but some of the gums, oils and spices they mention are expensive and very difficult to obtain. Orris powder 'fixes' or holds the perfumes of the other ingredients; and peel of oranges, lemons, tangerines or satsumas, dried in a cool oven until crisp, then put through a grinder and added to the mixture, will also act as a fixing agent.

Pot pourri should not have a heavy scent, but a light elusive perfume needing just a stir of the hand to refresh it. It is pleasant to have it in open bowls in a room, but it will keep its colour and fragrance longer if it can be stored in a covered jar.

Above right: A selection of dried flowers and scented herbs suitable for pot pourri.
Below right: Flower petals, herbs, oils and spices being assembled in preparation for making a pot pourri mixture.

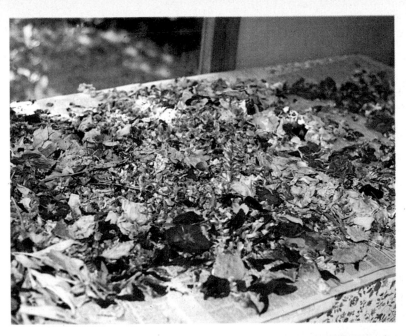

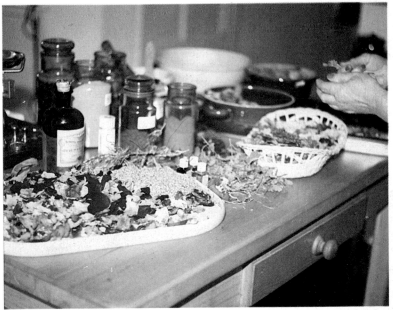

LEAF SHAPES

1   2   3   4   5   6

1. lanceolate
2. oblanceolate
3. ovate
4. obovate
5. elliptic
6. linear
7. cordate
8. reniform

7   8

LEAF MARGINS

entire   serrate   crenate   lobed

FLOWER ARRANGEMENTS

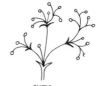

spike   raceme   panicle   cyme

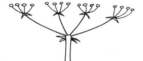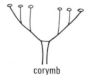

umbels (making a compound umbel)   corymb

About this Book

The herbs described in this book grow wild or can be cultivated in northern Europe, and many are commonly known in North America, Australasia and other parts of the world. Even between northern and southern Britain there are variations in weather patterns, so a general guide to the seasons in which plants flower is given rather than specific months. Soil and climatic conditions affect the ultimate size to which plants grow so the heights should be taken as an approximate guide.

The herbs are grouped alphabetically in botanical families, the common name first, then the genus and species in Latin. If we take Peppermint as an example: the family is Labiateae (with lipped flowers), the genus is *Mentha* (mint) and the species *piperita* (with a peppery, hot taste). Common names vary from one place to another but Latin names are adopted internationally, so a knowledge of the latter makes identification of plants easier and more positive. The glossary below explains some of the Latin words used to describe species:

acetosa: acid
alba: white
angustifolia: narrow-leaved
aquatica: growing in or near water
aureus: golden
balsamita: balsam-scented
chamaecyparissus: ground cypress-like
chenopodium: leaves of goose-foot shape
citriodorus: lemon-scented
crispum: curled
didyma: in pairs
dioica: male and female flowers on separate plants
erythreae: pink or red
fistulosum: hollow or pipe-like stems
foetidus: foetid smelling, stinking
glabrous: hairless
glaucous: blue-green
graveolens: strong-smelling
hederaceous: ivy-like
hortensis: of the garden
icterina: jaundice-yellow
incana: white or hoary
lactiflora: milky-white flowers
lanuginosus: woolly or downy
lappa: with burs
lateriflora: flowers arranged on one side of flower stalk
laterifolius: leaves arranged on one side of stem
longifolius: long-leaved
maculatus: spotted or blotched
millefolium: finely divided leaves
mollis: soft or velvety
montanus: growing on mountains
moschata: smelling of musk

nana: dwarf
napellus: turnip-rooted
nigra: black
odoratus: fragrant
oleracea: eaten as cultivated herb
orientalis: eastern, of the Orient
perenne: lasting through the year
petiolata: having petioles; leaf stalks
planum: flat
pubescens: softly hairy or downy
pulegium: from Latin *pulex*, flea (to be used against fleas)
pratensis: of meadowland
punctata: dotted with spots or glands
purpurascens: purplish
reptans: creeping
rosulatus: in a rosette
rotundifolia: round-leaved
rubiginosa: rust-red
sativum: cultivated
scutatus: shield-shaped
sempervirens: green throughout year
sericea: clothed with silky hairs
serpyllum: creeping
serrulatus: finely saw-toothed
spicatus: spiked
splendens: shining or gleaming
suaveolens: sweetly scented
sylvestris: of the wood, wild
tinctoria: a dye plant
tricolor: three-coloured
usitatissimum: very common
ulmaria: elm-like leaves
variegatus: with variegated leaves
vera: true
viridis or *virens:* green
vulgaris: common or ordinary

HERB FAMILIES

Family Acanthaceae

ACANTHUS
(Bear's Breeches, Thorn Flower)
Acanthus mollis
This hardy perennial has spreading, fleshy roots, with a dense growth of hollow-stemmed, deeply lobed, bright green leaves (40–50cm long) shooting directly from the roots. Soft hairs give a sheen to their surfaces. Its creamy-white flowers, streaked with pink and green, are borne on stiff spikes up to 150cm high. The flowers are 5cm long, with a deeply divided, prominent front petal and a leafy calyx which varies from green to purple. There is a protective sepal behind the petal, and small, sharply-spiked leaflets in front. Flowers midsummer to autumn.

Cultivation: will grow in sun or shade in most soils; looks well against a dark background or as a feature plant in island beds. Once established is best left undisturbed, though it may be necessary to remove young plants growing from roots spreading beyond alloted area. Transplant in spring or autumn. If grown from seed, may take 3–4 years to flower.

Uses: an emollient herb once used to soothe burns and sore joints. The beauty of the acanthus leaf inspired the decorative leaf work on Corinthian pillars which has been copied over the centuries. The leaves also feature on a 10th-century stole, now in Durham cathedral, which was embroidered in memory of St Cuthbert within 15 years of the death of King Alfred the Great. *Acanthus spinosus* is a smaller plant with leaves sharply divided giving a spiky effect.

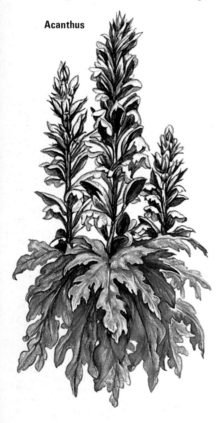

Acanthus

Family Boraginaceae

ALKANET
(Evergreen Alkanet)
Pentaglottis sempervirens
A persistent hardy perennial (to 65cm) which remains in leaf during the winter. Its root is thick, branching and dark-skinned. The pointed, ovate leaves are up to 32cm long and 15cm wide, with a noticeable network of veins. Both the stalk and the leaves are hairy. The rich blue flowers, like large forget-me-nots, are arranged on one side of short spikes and bloom from late spring to autumn. The fresh green foliage is welcome in winter, but the plant spreads rapidly and is best in informal settings.

Cultivation: plant in spring or autumn. Will tolerate sun or shade and most soils. First flowering shoots should be cut down when they wither to stimulate healthy new growth (this surplus material can be used for mulching during dry weather provided the ground is well soaked first). To propagate, cut thick roots into pieces 10cm long, place in drill and cover with 8–10cm of good soil. In spring young leaves can be confused with those of comfrey *(Symphytum officinalis)*, which are edible. Alkanet leaves should not be eaten because they may contain poisonous alkaloids. The surface leaf hairs are softer than those of comfrey, giving a slight shine. Later in the year, comparison of the flowers will avoid any error.

Uses: a red dye, extracted from alkanet and its close relative *Anchusa officinalis*, is included in a list of simples used by Hippocrates, the father of medicine, who practised his skills four hundred years before the birth of Christ. The colour was used as a cosmetic by women in ancient Egypt and in oils for medication and dyes for fabrics over the centuries.

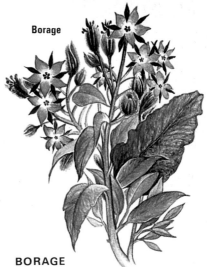

Borage

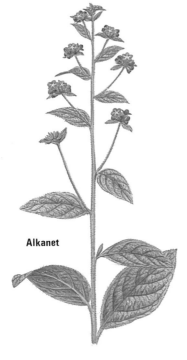

Alkanet

BORAGE
(Burrage)
Borago officinalis
A hardy annual, sometimes biennial, covered with stiff hairs making it rough to the touch. It has a branching taproot, and the stem grows 50–60cm high. The ovate leaves (20 x 10cm) are deeply veined, and the vivid blue, starlike flowers have 5 pointed petals, prominent erect black stamens, and a reddish calyx. There is also a white-flowered variety.

Cultivation: easily grown where it is required to flower from spring-sown seed, but does not transplant well. Usually produces robust self-sown seedlings in subsequent years.

Uses: for those who find cucumber indigestible, borage gives flavour without causing discomfort. If the hairy skin is peeled from young stalks, the succulent inside may be chopped into salads. The flowers are also edible, and are used with the small leaves to give a cool flavour to summer drinks. The beauty of its flowers made borage a popular subject for embroidery, sometimes also showing the bees for whom it is a favourite herb. It can be used as a poultice for external inflammation, and may be beneficial if taken as a tea by those with rheumatic tendencies.

21

Lungwort

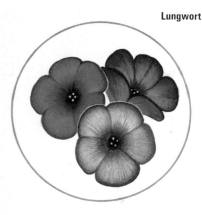

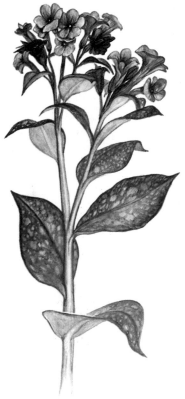

LUNGWORT
(Soldiers & Sailors, Jerusalem Cowslip)
Pulmonaria officinalis
A hardy herb dying down in winter; early in spring dense basal growth shoots from the creeping rootstock. The ovate leaves (15 x 8cm) and the stems (to 30cm) are hairy and rough to the touch. The foliage shows irregular white blotches and the flower stalks often display blooms of two colours at the same time, deep pink to red and purple or blue. The cowslip-like tubular flowers ($1\frac{1}{2}$cm) are arranged in short terminal cymes. Lungwort is usually one of the first herbs to flower in early spring.

Cultivation: autumn is the best time to lift and divide roots, thereby avoiding disturbance when the plant is coming into flower in spring. The roots, from which young leaf growth can be seen shooting, should be cut into 6–8cm pieces. Trim off the old leaves and plant in a fairly moist, semi-shady position. Lungwort will provide useful ground cover and, if the flower stalks are cut back as they wither, the spotted leaves will continue to give interest until they die in winter.

Uses: in the 16th century a theory known as the Doctrine of Signatures was expounded by the herbalist and physician , Paracelsus, contending that plants are marked in particular ways in their colour or form to indicate how they are beneficial. The spotted lung-shaped leaves of lungwort pointed to its use for diseases of the lungs and the Latin name *Pulmonaria officinalis* (official herb for pulmonary complaints) established it until recently as a treatment for certain chest ailments. It also served as a pot herb and as a vegetable. Because of their generous and cheerful habit of early flowering, other lungworts are worth acquiring. *P. angustifolia* has deep azure-blue flowers, and the white-flowered variety *P. alba* is a good foil to spring bulbs.

COMMON COMFREY
(Knitbone, Bruisewort)
Symphytum officinalis

A strong-growing hardy perennial dying down in winter. The plant (50–100cm) develops from the basal leaf growth up squared and flattened hollow stems with pointed ovate deeply-veined leaves decreasing in size from 40 x 15cm at ground level to 4–6cm under the flower clusters. Leaves are alternate and the bell-shaped tubular flowers, in bloom late spring to autumn, are arranged on one side of the stem. They are usually creamy-white but pink and mauve variants exist. In spring when only the basal leaves have grown they can be confused with the foxglove's. But comfrey leaves when crushed have a smell of cucumber and if the back of the leaf is brushed across the back of the hand its rough scratching hairs can be felt. Foxglove leaves are also hairy, but soft to the touch, and they should never be eaten.

Cultivation: it is so easy to increase comfrey from root cuttings that it is not worth trying to grow it from seed. In spring and autumn roots may be cut into short pieces, laid horizontally in drills and then covered with 5–8cm of good soil. Because comfrey produces so much leaf growth it does best in deep moist soil. Left undisturbed it will spread rapidly so it is wise to plant it in an area where the rampant growth will be welcome.

Uses: Comfrey is a valuable plant which has proved its worth over hundreds of years. Its common names reflect its reputation for helping bones to knit and soothing bruises. The root contains allantoin which encourages healthy cell growth, mucilage which soothes, protein (unusual in plant material) and vitamin B12. The root or leaves, crushed and applied as a poultice, will usually relieve external inflammation and may be taken as a tea to ease internal inflammation. Comfrey ointment applied to burns, sprains and strains, bruises and aching limbs will often give quick relief, but the rough hairy leaves should never be applied

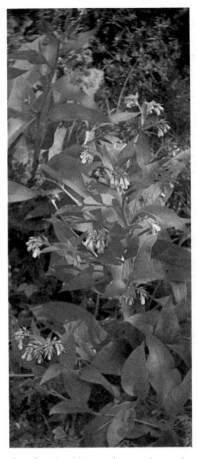

Comfrey is a vigorously growing and useful herb.

directly to the skin because they can act as an irritant. The peeled roots chopped into chunks and the young leaves cooked like spinach make acceptable vegetable dishes. In the garden the big leaves can be roughly chopped with a spade and laid at the bottom of trenches for celery or under plantings of potatoes, peas, beans etc. Comfrey makes good compost and mulch.

23

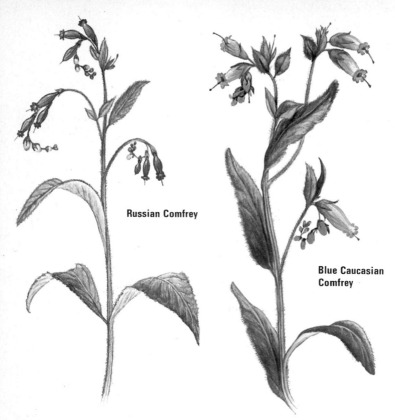

Russian Comfrey

Blue Caucasian Comfrey

RUSSIAN COMFREY
Symphytum x uplandicum
A tough, strong-growing perennial with thick spreading roots which dies down in winter. The stems (to 120cm) bear leaves 40–50cm long with raised midribs on their undersides and crinkled edges which tend to turn inwards towards the centre. The flowers are deep violet-blue.
Cultivation: the same as that of common comfrey.
Uses: Russian comfrey is a valuable fodder crop and is also used in the garden for composting and mulching. It should not be grown in borders as a decorative plant as it is too vigorous. Only the fresh young leaves are taken for culinary use and if the plant is cut back as growth matures it will soon produce new foliage.

BLUE CAUCASIAN COMFREY
Symphytum Caucasicum
This attractive member of the family is easy to grow. The leaves (20 x 8cm) are not so roughly hairy as those of common and Russian comfrey and in spring the plant grows into a neat cone shape with tight clusters of sky-blue flowers.
Cultivation: by root cuttings as with common comfrey. This cultivar seeds freely and young plants will be found coming up around the parent plant after the first season.
Uses: can be included with spring-flowering subjects in a herbaceous border and if cut down when the first flower stems have withered will make another pleasant display in August–September. The young leaves can be used in salads.

SOFT COMFREY
Symphytum orientale
Similar in growth to Caucasian comfrey but the broader, more oval leaves (19 x 9cm) are noticeably softer to the touch than those of the other comfreys. The short tubular flowers are more rounded and always white.

Cultivation: by root cuttings. All the comfreys have dark or black skinned branching roots which when peeled reveal a cream-coloured fleshy interior. The hairy leaves and arrangement of the flowers as a curled nodding terminal cyme are characteristic of these herbs.

Uses: the light green foliage and pure white bell flowers and its compact, bushy habit make this comfrey acceptable in a herb border, a good foil for plants with pink, mauve or blue flowers, the early spring plumes of bronze fennel or the blue-green foliage of Jackman's blue rue.

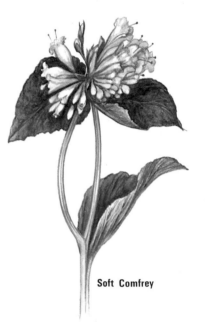

Soft Comfrey

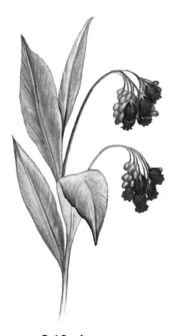

Red Comfrey

RED COMFREY
Symphytum rubrum
This crimson-flowered hybrid is not very robust and should be grown in soil containing plenty of humus so that it does not dry out. It needs moisture so a position in semi-shade is best. It seldom grows to more than 30cm and comes into flower later than the other comfreys, from July onwards. It is not invasive and will flower on into the autumn attracting attention by the rich colour of its blooms.

Cultivation: this less-common and attractive comfrey is propagated, like the others, by root cuttings, but it is worthwhile starting them off in boxes of good compost and taking care to protect the young shoots from slugs. Take the same precautions when the plants are moved to their permanent site.

Uses: a good plant to grow near lungwort in semi-shade, providing colour later in the season.

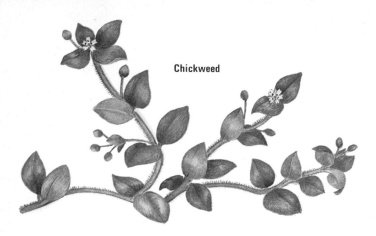

Chickweed

Family Caryophyllaceae

CHICKWEED
(Starweed)
Stellaria media
A persistent common annual herb with weak sprawling stems which are hairy

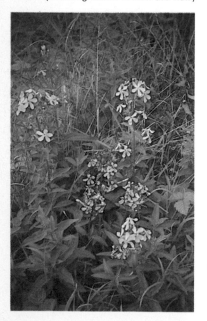

on one side only. The pale green pointed oval leaves grow in opposite pairs, almost hiding the tiny white flowers (5–7mm) which have 5 deeply cleft petals and narrow sepals of the same length making a star formation. The fruits are projected on elongated drooping stalks.

Cultivation: if allowed to grow on a small damp unwanted piece of ground it will seed freely, propagating itself throughout the year.

Uses: it is easy to underestimate a plant most gardeners regard as a troublesome weed, but this herb will provide tasty salad material, even in winter, with a slightly salty, nutty flavour. If it grows in abundance it may be cooked like spinach as a vegetable: wash the leaves and cook in just the water adhering to them, adding a knob of butter and boiling in a covered saucepan over a gentle heat for 5–7 minutes. Before serving, grate a little nutmeg or finely chop some chives over it. Chickweed has a cool soothing effect on the skin and is crushed and applied fresh as a poultice or used in ointments for burns, rashes and to ease the pain of aching joints. It is a favourite food of small birds; because of its ability to propagate itself, the seeds provide valuable winter feed for them.

The roots and leaves of soapwort can be used instead of shampoo to cleanse the hair with a gentle action.

SOAPWORT
(Latherwort, Bouncing Bet)
Saponaria officinalis
A hairless perennial with spreading rootstock. The stiff, smoothly-ridged stems (50–75cm) are pale green, sometimes with a red tinge. The oval pointed leaves (5–7cm) with ribbed veins are arranged in opposite pairs growing from swollen leaf joints. The pink flowers are either 5-petalled and single or many-petalled and double. Enclosed in a tubular calyx, they grow in terminal clusters in late summer and have the sweet clove scent typical of the pink family.
Cultivation: Soapwort does not grow reliably from seed but may be easily propagated in spring from pieces of creeping root showing young leaf buds. Damp friable soil will encourage growth and the name Bouncing Bet reflects the freedom with which the plants grow in a favourable situation.
Uses: this plant has served as a natural soap, probably for thousands of years, for cleansing woollens, silks and many beautiful fabrics. In modern times its gentle cleansing action has been successfully used to freshen and restore the colours of old tapestries.

Family Caprifoliaceae

ELDER
(Pipe tree)
Sambucus nigra
A large deciduous shrub or small tree (10–12m) distinguished by its flat heads of creamy flowers in June and purple-black berries in autumn. The dull green leaves, arranged as 5 leaflets with serrated edges, take on a pinkish tinge when the berries ripen.
Cultivation: strikes easily from hardwood cuttings pulled off with a heel in spring, cut to 14cm and inserted 7cm into sandy compost. The tree does well on heavy soil.
Uses: few small trees have so much folklore connected with them; Mother Elder was said to protect the garden and its occupants, and in parts of the country people are still reluctant to cut down an elder. Around 400 BC, the elder was included in Hippocrates' list of important plants and it has been in constant use up to modern times for such diverse purposes as children's pea shooters, musical pipes, wines, conserves, cosmetics and cures.

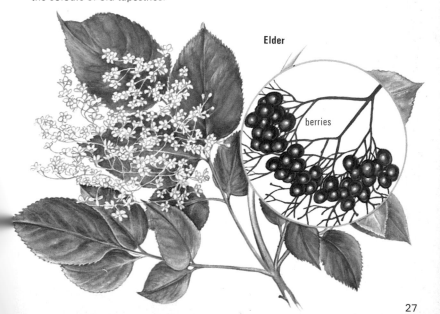

Elder

berries

Family Compositeae

ALECOST
(Costmary, Bible leaf)
Chrysanthemum balsamita tanacetoides
A hardy perennial dying back in winter. In spring clumps of fresh green leaves come from the woody stems lying horizontally just below the surface of the soil. The herb grows into a loosely bushy plant up to 100cm with light green leaves (6–12cm) roundly toothed at the edges. The flowers are in flat clusters of yellow disc florets, similar to but smaller than those of tansy.

Cultivation: in northern Europe this herb is difficult to grow from seed but it is easily propagated by pulling off young rooted pieces of basal stem in spring. It spreads rapidly and becomes straggly and untidy, so it is wise to discard old plants every 3–4 years and start again from young stock.

Uses: in the past, alecost was one of the herbs with antiseptic properties strewn on the floor in crowded dwellings to purify the air. It was also put between bedding and clothing to impart a fresh smell and was used to· flavour ales. With the revival of 'real ale'

it may be of interest again. It is bitter in taste but the leaves when crushed smell of mint and when very young may be used sparingly in salads. Its common name 'bible leaf' may come from it being used as a bookmark in church bibles. In the days when sermons were very long, its refreshing scent must have been welcome.

CAMPHOR PLANT
Balsamita vulgaris
Camphor is similar to alecost in all its growing habits, but may be distinguished by the colour of its leaves which are a greyer green and its flowers, like small daisies, with white ray florets and yellow disc floret centres.

Cultivation: the same as alecost.

Uses: the camphor plant smells strongly of camphor oil which comes from the tree *Cinnamonum camphora*, not hardy in this country. Put among linen, furs and woollens its familiar mothball smell discourages moths. But it can also be dried and mixed with lavender and southernwood, in equal quantities, to make a sweeter-smelling mixture. It is one of the less common herbs.

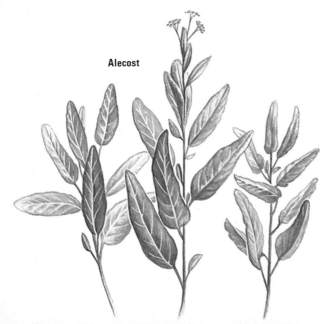

Alecost

BURDOCK, COMMON & BURDOCK, GREATER

Arctium minus & Arctium lappa

These sturdy biennials share the same characteristics of large downy leaves and round heads of burs. The strong taproots penetrate deeply into the waste ground where the plants are often seen growing wild and the stiff branching stems grow to 70–90cm. The coarse textured leaves, sometimes over 30cm long at the base of the plant, are arranged alternately and decrease in size up the stem. They are broadly ovate and pointed at the tips, with downy undersides. The leaves of the greater burdock are rounder at the tips and the stalks are furrowed on the upper surface. The egg-shaped buds open to show purple florets, which, together with shorter, sepal-like, hooked bracts, form the burs in late summer. One common name for burdock, Happy Major, may have originated from the burs being used as buttons to transform, in imagination, a child's plain clothing into a smart-looking uniform.

Cultivation: if burdock is introduced into the garden it should be kept apart from any designed herb planting as it seeds freely and will become invasive. If required for edible or medicinal use, it is best planted in a deep, well-drained soil in which it will produce good straight roots.

Uses: this plant was included in Hippocrates' list of useful plants. It has been found to contain antibiotic substances which aid resistance to infection and can help to cure skin complaints. A decoction is made from 1-year-old roots which have been washed and scraped. Chop 30gr (1oz) of root and add to 0.85 litre (1½ pints) of cold water which is slowly brought to the boil then allowed to simmer until it reduces to 0.5 litre (1 pint). The mucilage in the root will slightly thicken the decoction which can be drunk and also used to bathe the skin. In spring, country people whose diet had been deficient in vitamins over the winter months used to make a drink made from burdock and dandelion roots which acted as a blood purifier and cleared up skin troubles. The very young stalks may be peeled and chopped into salads and later can be cooked as a vegetable.

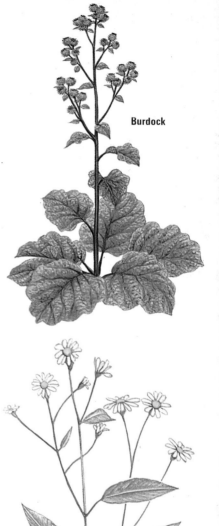

Burdock

Camphor plant

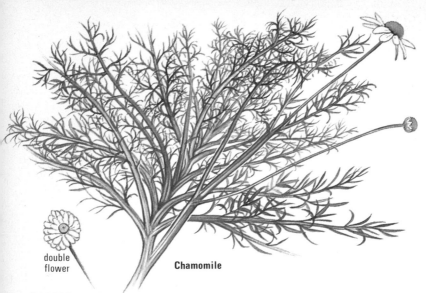

double
flower

Chamomile

CHAMOMILE
(Ground Apple, Roman chamomile)
Chamaemelum nobile (Anthemis nobilis)
Chamomile plants can have single, double or no flowers. It is perennial, prostrate or low-growing, with short fibrous spreading roots. The bright green leaves are very finely divided and the plant has a pleasant apple scent, especially when bruised or trodden on. Single flowers have a yellow disc and white ray florets, double flowers are cream-coloured and the yellow disc is not evident.

Cultivation: single-flowered chamomile can be grown from seed in spring. Sow the tiny seeds very thinly in boxes or trays and prick out the seedlings when they are big enough to handle. The young plantlets should be set 15cm apart in their permanent positions. This is an economical method of raising a quantity of plants, but if they are used for lawn-making quite frequent mowing will be necessary to prevent them becoming straggly. Double flowered chamomile should be propagated by pulling off young rooted plantlets from the parent at the end of May or in September. Non-flowering chamomile, now known as 'Treneague', is the best one to make into fragrant paths, small lawns or a mossy looking 'mat' in front of a garden seat or around a sundial, bird-bath or other garden ornament. The young plantlets should be set out on clean ground 15cm apart in staggered rows and made very firm. They will spread out, filling in the spaces between them. Rolling helps to establish the new roots and all weeds should be removed by hand as soon as they appear; selective weed-killers will destroy the chamomile. When the lawn is established it will need mowing a couple of times during the summer to keep it compact and stimulate new growth. German chamomile *Chamomilla recutita, (Matricaria chamomilla)* is an annual single-flowered variety, similar to the single perennial Roman chamomile but growing to 30cm.

Uses: one of the most beneficial of herb teas, chamomile was recommended for headaches, chills, fevers, digestive trouble, as a fomentation for swellings, for nervous conditions and as a tonic to brighten fair hair. For a pint of chamomile tea allow 6 flowers, infuse for 5–10 minutes and, if liked, add a small teaspoonful of honey to each cup.

CHICORY
(Succory)
Cichorium intybus
A perennial with a parsnip-like taproot and a stiff rather hairy stem (50–100cm). The leaves first form a rosette at the base of the stem, then diminish in size, deeply cut like dandelions, alternately up the stem. The unstalked flowers are usually in pairs, with ray florets only. They are bright sky-blue in the mornings but fade from midday. Chicory and evening primrose are a good combination as the latter's flowers open in late afternoon.

Cultivation and uses: easily grown from seed thinly sown out of doors in late spring; the Witloof variety is best for salads. Plant the seedlings 8cm apart in a circle and cover them with a large plastic bucket to blanch the leaves. Green unblanched leaves are coarse, woolly and bitter. To force chicory for winter salads, set the plants in rows and earth them up like potatoes in September, ensuring that the ridge is at least 15cm over the trimmed crowns of the roots. Magdeburg chicory produces good roots which can be dug, scraped, roasted in shallow trays in the oven and then ground as a coffee substitute. The rather bitter flavour can be neutralized by adding honey.

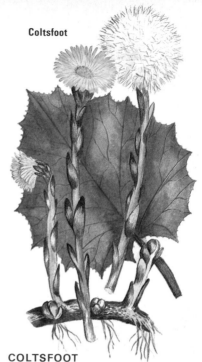

Coltsfoot

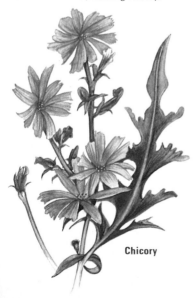

Chicory

COLTSFOOT
(Son-before-Father)
Tussilago farfara
Herb with creeping rootstock and net-veined, broadly heart-shaped leaves with edges toothed and undersides covered with cottony down. It is the shape of the leaves , some of which grow 25–30cm across, which gives the plant its name. The flowers, like small dandelions (2–3cm), are borne singly on reddish scaly fleshy stems. They appear in spring before the leaves, hence the name Son-before-Father.

Cultivation: can be grown from seed gathered from the flower 'clocks' or from pieces of root detached from a plant. Coltsfoot is a vigorous, rampant grower and should be confined to waste patches in the garden.

Uses: one of the most valuable herbs for coughs and chest complaints. It is an important ingredient of the herbal tobacco smoked by sufferers from respiratory disorders and can be made into a soothing drink for troublesome coughs.

31

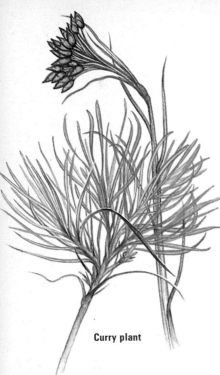

Curry plant

Uses: these are decorative and interesting plants rather than useful herbs from a culinary point of view. The leaves cannot be used to make curry despite their appetising smell. They are bitter to taste and although they may be used with discretion it should be as a garnish rather than as a flavouring. For those interested in silver foliage plants another species is worth mentioning, *Helichrysum alveolatum*. Similar in habit and size to those just described, this bush has shorter, narrow, woolly-looking leaves ($1\frac{1}{2}$cm), forming a close tuft at the top of the stem. Flowers appear in autumn and make a cheerful golden display through the winter.

DANDELION
(Lion's tooth, Priest's crown)
Taraxacum officinale
A common, widely distributed perennial herb with a strong taproot. The irregularly jagged toothed leaves in the basal rosette vary in shape and are lanceolate with a grooved central vein which directs rain to the root through the centre of the rosette. The flowers, borne singly on hollow stems, are

CURRY PLANT
Helichrysum angustifolium & H. plicatum
Two closely related bushy perennial herbs with soft hairs covering the stems and leaves, giving the plants a silvery appearance. *H. plicatum* is a little more grey-silver and appears to withstand winter weather better. They grow to bushes approximately 50cm tall and 60cm across and on both the leaves (5cm) are linear. When any part of the bushes are touched the curry smell is immediately evident. The flowers are in small flat heads of golden yellow disc florets, rather like miniature tansy flowers.
Cultivation: by cuttings in spring or autumn. A sunny, well-drained, open position is best. As the plant grows any wayward branches should be removed as they may otherwise split out from the centre of the bush.

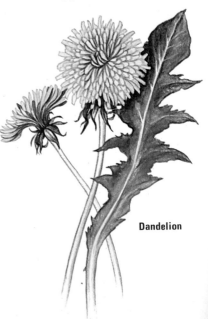

Dandelion

composed only of ray florets maturing to the familiar dandelion 'clock', whose windborne seeds, each with its own parachute, ensure continuity.

Cultivation: by seed sown in spring. If bigger, less toothed leaves are wanted, it is possible to obtain seed of a cultivated variety of dandelion. All dandelion leaves are slightly bitter, the young ones less so, but much of the bitterness can be removed by blanching. This is done by covering the plants to exclude the light with large flat stones, strong lightproof boxes, flower pots, plastic buckets or sheets of black or blue polythene. Precautions should be taken to prevent slugs eating the succulent blanched growth.

Uses: the dandelion is one of the most valuable of all known herbs, having more uses and medicinal properties than many cultivated vegetables. Dandelion coffee made from roots washed, scraped, roasted and ground, is the best substitute for true coffee. The white latex juice from the roots and stems was used in the treatment of warts and moles. The leaves contain vitamins A, B and C. Not only are they good in salads but help to stimulate the appetite, act as a mild laxative, are an effective diuretic, and provide relief from dyspepsia, liver disorders and some rheumatic conditions. The herb is safe to take in any quantity. Dandelion wine is one of the best-known country wines. With the abundance of flowers in spring it is easy to collect material for winemaking, though roadsides where the flowers have been subjected to traffic fumes should be avoided.

ELECAMPANE
(Scabwort)
Inula Helenium
A handsome tall-growing perennial dying down in winter. The thick taproot (15–20cm long) can be 10–15cm across at the crown when mature. In spring the root produces rosettes of basal leaves growing 20–40cm long and 12–15cm across, pointed ovate with undersides covered with downy hairs. The stiff, hairy stems ($1\frac{1}{2}$–2m) bear alternate stalkless leaves which diminish in size as they reach the cluster of yellow flowers. These open in succession, showing a single row of ray

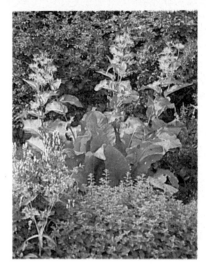

Elecampane makes a handsome plant at the back of a herb bed.

florets which droop as the flowers fade. In bloom from midsummer, they are not unlike small sunflowers in appearance.

Cultivation: may be grown from seed sown in spring or when it is ripe in autumn. Easily propagated at these times by cutting off pieces of root bearing a bud or 'eye'. Requires moisture because of its large leaves and vigorous growth, so some compost and peat should be added to a light soil and a position in semi-shade chosen; on heavy moisture-retaining soil it will flourish in full sun. Soon after all the flowers have finished the stems grow woody and the herb looks bedraggled, so remove old stems and leaves.

Uses: this worthy herb has long been cultivated in this country. It grows in Europe, temperate Asia and N. America and is a valued treatment for coughs and other chest complaints, and for skin diseases in humans and animals (the origin of its common names 'scabwort' and 'horseheal'). It was candied as a pleasant sweetmeat with an aromatic pungent flavour said to 'help the digestion and cause mirth'. There are many legends associated with elecampane, one being that Helen of Troy was gathering it when she was carried off by Paris.

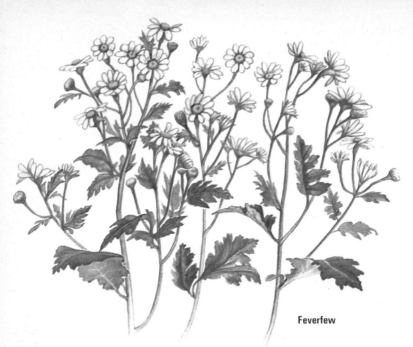

Feverfew

FEVERFEW
(Featherfew)
Chrysanthemum parthenium
Hardy short-lived perennial with many branching stems coming from the fibrous root and forming a compact bushy plant (45cm high and about the same across). The lime green leaves (5–7cm), composed of pinnate leaflets (1–1½cm), have serrated edges. The single flowers, which have a yellow disc and white ray florets, 1–2cm across, bloom from summer to autumn. Cultivated feverfew, or bachelors' buttons, has creamy-white double flowers with ray florets (1–2½cm).

Cultivation: feverfew grows freely from seed and will flourish in sun or shade on shallow well-drained soil; the seed can be sown in spring or early autumn. Plants grown from seed of the double variety may revert to single flowers. At most times of the year, when the weather is suitable, cuttings can be pulled off with a 'heel' from the base of the plant and set in sandy compost.

Uses: the names feverfew and featherfew may be corruptions of 'febrifuge', a term used to describe a herb employed to treat chills and fevers. When feverfew is found wild it is often near old cottages or in farmyards as it was thought that it could purify the atmosphere and help to ward off infection. An infusion of the leaves or flowers was taken to cure nervous headaches, to improve digestion and as a general tonic. Modern research has established the value of feverfew in the treatment of migraine. It is recommended that three leaves should be taken daily in a sandwich or chopped and added to food. It may also be of benefit in the treatment of some arthritic conditions.

GOLDEN FEVERFEW
(Golden Feather)
Chrysanthemum parthenium aureum
This herb is similar to the green-leaved feverfew, with the separate plants bearing single or double flowers, but its leaves are a bright golden colour and it makes an attractive foliage plant especially in winter when it provides a cheerful patch of colour.

HEMP AGRIMONY

Eupatorium cannabinum

A tall handsome perennial (up to 150cm high) with woody rootstock from which rise round, reddish, hairy branching stems. The stalked basal leaves are divided into 3, sometimes 5 lance-shaped lobes, the central one longer than the others; the stem leaves are scarcely stalked and those on the branches are undivided. The rosy pink flowerhead, a cyme formed of many small clusters of densely grouped florets, is in bloom from late summer.

Cultivation: by seed sown in spring or late summer or by root division. The plant appreciates a moisture-retaining soil in an open sunny position.

Uses: despite its name the only connection this herb has with hemp, *Cannabis sativa* (from which the drug cannabis is extracted), is the similarity in the shape of its leaves. It makes a good subject for the back of a border and continues to give interest when the flowerheads become a fluffy pappus of seeds with their little parachutes.

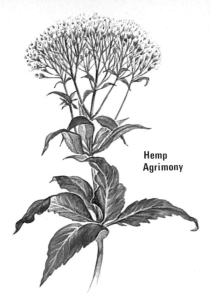

Hemp Agrimony

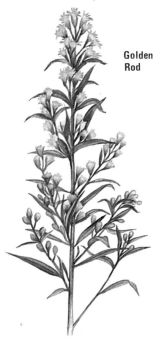

Golden Rod

GOLDEN ROD

Solidago virgaurea

An erect perennial with a dense growth of smooth or slightly hairy stems coming from rhizomes. Varies in size from 5cm on rocky or cliffside areas to 90–100cm on hedgebanks or dry open woodland. The lanceolate finely-toothed leaves are arranged alternately up the stems. On the upper part of the stem, branching flower stalks spring from the axils of the leaves and form a terminal panicle of small golden yellow flowers (10cm across) with a few disc and ray florets. The lower part of the flower is encased in green sepal-like bracts.

Cultivation: from pieces of rhizome pulled off at soil level in spring and set in good compost. Golden rod is particularly responsive to the quality of the soil in which it is grown and has a pleasant fragrance when it blooms from midsummer into autumn; it is a vigorous grower and should not be allowed to spread too far.

Uses: as its generic name which comes from *solidare* (to consolidate or make whole) indicates, golden rod has a reputation for healing wounds when applied as a poultice or used as an infusion to bathe the wound.

MARIGOLD
(Pot Marigold)
Calendula officinalis
A hardy annual (up to 50cm) familiar in many gardens because it seeds ·freely year after year. It has a fleshy white taproot and juicy stems branching at angles, with stalkless, lanceolate, slightly hairy leaves (up to 15cm) which are sticky to the touch. The single orange flowers have disc and ray florets up to 10cm across. In bloom for much of the year, its Latin name *calendula* testifies to its presence 'throughout the months'.
Cultivation: marigolds germinate quickly from spring sown seed. Seed sown in autumn will survive in poor conditions, but spring sowing makes healthier plants on good soil. Allow at least 30cm between each seedling so that the plants have room to develop if a good crop of leaves and flowers is to be harvested for drying. The hard curved seeds, sometimes 1cm long, look curiously like petrified grubs. The flowers will come into bloom in quick succession and need picking every day or so. The outer ray 'petals' (florets) are stripped off the disc, spread thinly on sieves and placed in a warm place in the dark (see page 14). The petals should be lightly tossed with the fingers every day to ensure even drying, and then stored in air-tight containers out of the light. In this way, they will keep their bright orange colour.
Uses: Calendula has an ancient history and has proved of considerable importance in the treatment of many skin complaints because of its antiseptic and anti-inflammatory properties. Both leaves and flowers are used and affected parts are bathed with an infusion or dressed with an ointment or lotion made from the plant. The juice can be expressed from the leaves and applied directly to the skin. It is used for ulcers and other inflamed areas and can be taken internally as a tea. The flowers yield a good orange dye which one of the old herbalists suggests was once used to colour the hair of those 'not content with the colour God had given them'. The name pot marigold has nothing to do with the plant being grown in a pot but is a corruption of the word 'pottage', indicating its use in

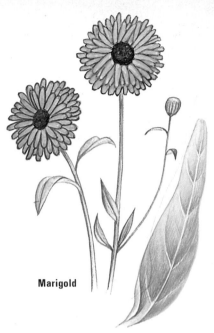

Marigold

soups and stews. It makes a wholesome colouring agent for cheese, and the young leaves and flowers are used in salads and are a good substitute for saffron in rice for buns and cakes.
Dyeing: marigold yields an orange dye, golden rod a lemon-yellow one. Both should be used with a mordant (fixative) made of alum. To experiment with 110gr (4oz) wool, take 230gr ($\frac{1}{2}$lb) flowering tops, cut them up and put them in a pot with enough water to cover. Bring slowly to the boil and simmer gently for an hour or so; remove from heat and cool. For the mordant, dissolve 30gr (1oz) alum and 10gr ($\frac{1}{4}$oz) tartaric acid in 0.30 litre ($\frac{1}{2}$pt) boiling water; add this to 2.25 litres ($\frac{1}{2}$ gallon) of soft water in a pot and let it warm. Soak the wool thoroughly in a bowl of water with a pinch of washing soda added, then remove it and slip it into the mordant solution. Bring to the boil, then simmer slowly for at least an hour. Heat the dye solution to simmering point, strain and transfer the wool from the mordant to the dye pot. Simmer until the required colour is

obtained; remove the pot from the heat and let it cool, leaving the wool in the pot. When cold remove the wool and rinse it thoroughly several times until no colour comes out. Squeeze away the surplus moisture but do not wring, then hang the wool in an airy place to dry. Chamomile, dandelion, hop and elder are a few other herbs which can be used for dyeing. There are endless combinations of natural materials and various mordants which can be used.

"MACE"
(Nutmeg Thyme)
Achillea decolorans
A less common, pleasing perennial herb (to 35cm) which dies down in winter. Fibrous roots form a clump from which grow stems bearing alternate linear fine-toothed leaves (5cm). The flowers are in terminal clusters with creamy-white ray and short disc florets (1cm across).
Cultivation: from division of root in spring when small pieces may be easily separated from the parent plant. It likes a well-drained sunny position and the clumps should be split and replanted every 3–4 years.

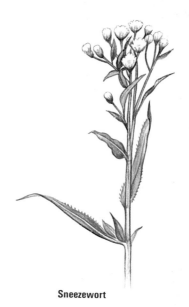

Sneezewort

Uses: the true mace is the webby aril around the nutmeg which is marketed as blade or ground mace. This herb gets its names of 'mace' and 'nutmeg thyme' because its smell is so similar to the true spice and it can be used instead of nutmeg or mace in cooking.

SNEEZEWORT
Achillea ptarmica
A bushy erect perennial (to 60cm) dying back in winter with dense stem growth and dark green, lanceolate, serrated leaves (8cm). It has clusters of true white double daisy-type flowers with ray florets and an insignificant central disc. Flowers from midsummer, opening a succession of flower clusters until autumn – a good foil for other colours.
Cultivation: by division of root in spring or autumn. Likes a rather moist position and will spread steadily. The root becomes densely entangled so it is wise to divide the clumps and replant every 3–4 years.
Uses: the name sneezewort indicates its use, when dried and powdered, as a snuff taken to clear the nasal passages.

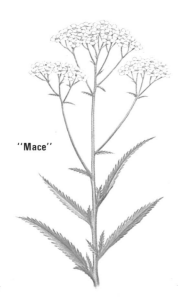

"Mace"

SOUTHERNWOOD
(Old Man, Lads Love)
Artemisia abrotanum

A woody perennial losing its leaves in winter. It forms a shrubby bush (to 100cm) which from spring through to late autumn is densely covered with fine thread-like leaves. The flowers are sometimes absent or so inconspicuous as to be hardly noticed but the aromatic smell from the foliage has made this herb a long time favourite cottage garden plant.

Cultivation: like many of the artemisias, southernwood does not grow well from seed in Britain but cuttings strike easily if taken in spring or late summer. It should be trimmed into shape each autumn to prevent the bushes getting straggly and ungainly.

Uses: this was one of the strewing herbs of olden days. When walked on, its wholesome scent helped to make unhygienic conditions more supportable. It was also given to children to expel worms, and put among clothes to discourage moths (which is the reason for its French name of garderobe). An infusion rubbed into the scalp was thought to stimulate the growth of hair. Rubbing any infusion on a hairless head will not make hair grow, but the massaging of the scalp with some herb infusions will have a healthy effect on existing hair. Dried southernwood can be added to pot pourri mixtures to give a lemony scent. Mixed with lavender or any of the fragrant mints and oatmeal, and made up in small muslin or cotton bags, it can be hung under the hot water tap to give fragrance to a bath and help to soften hard water.

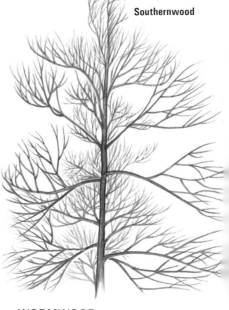

Southernwood

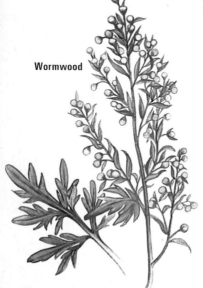

Wormwood

WORMWOOD
(Old Woman)
Artemisia absinthium

A woody perennial (to 90cm). The basal leaves are lobed and deeply divided; the stem leaves linear. All are covered with close silky hairs on their upper and lower surfaces, which gives the plant a silvered look. The flowers develop on the terminal and lateral stems as panicles of small yellow rayless blooms which look rather like mimosa.

Cultivation: from seed or cuttings in spring or late summer. The seed is minute and should be mixed with fine sand and the whole scattered thinly on top of the soil and not covered. There is a cultivar, Lambrook Silver, which makes more compact and dense silvery growth than the type and is the better one to grow in a herb bed. It should be propagated by cuttings or root division.

Uses: in the past, wormwood was administered to get rid of intestinal worms. An infusion made from it is drunk to settle a disturbed stomach, but the flavour is so intensely bitter – it is one of the bitterest herbs known – that it is not found acceptable by most people. As a silver foliage plant it is attractive.

SUNFLOWER
Helianthus annuus
A well-known annual producing plants from 50cm to 5m high. The round, rough erect stems carry ovate leaves (5–30cm) with toothed edges, and the solitary flowerheads, with golden ray and brown disc florets, can be anything from 7 to 30cm across.

Cultivation: from seed sown in pots or boxes indoors in April. The young plants must be put out when all danger of frost is past, or sown out of doors in May where they are to grow. The flowerhead is top heavy so support will be needed and a sheltered site is advised. Thought to be a native of Mexico this plant has been grown in many parts of the world as a valuable domestic and commercial commodity, the seed providing food for humans and animals, the leaves used for cattle food, the stem fibre employed in paper-making. Sunflower margarine is among the best of those high in poly-unsaturates and sunflower oil is an excellent substitute for olive oil in salads and cooking or herb oils for skin treatment.

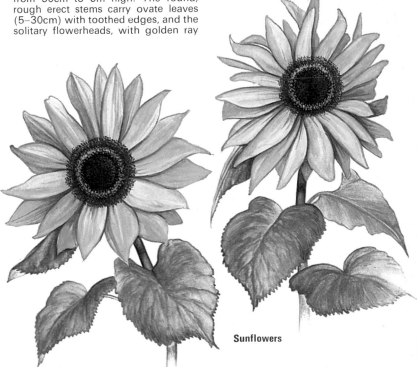

Sunflowers

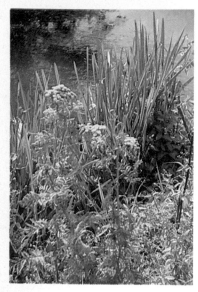

Tansy grows wild beside rivers, lakes and canals.

TANSY
(Buttons)
Tanacetum vulgare
An erect hardy perennial (to 120cm) on stiff stems with dark green, feathery, pinnate, irregularly toothed leaves, which are strongly aromatic. The flowers are corymbs of gold 'buttons', all disc florets, from midsummer.
Cultivation: by root division or pieces of rhizome pulled off in spring or autumn. Tansy, a vigorous herb to the point of becoming invasive, is best in an informal setting. It is an interesting-looking plant and could fill gaps between spring-flowering shrubs, its yellow flowerheads giving colour from summer through to autumn.
Uses: tansy cakes and tansy puddings were eaten during Lent and the herb is thought to have been one of the bitter herbs of the Passover. Bitter it certainly is and should be used with discretion in cooking. It excels at discouraging flies, and as it is often found by riversides can help fishermen to keep flies away from themselves and their catch. A few fresh leaves rubbed between the hands to bruise them and then tucked into clothing gives protection from flies when working or sitting in the garden. Bunches cut freshly each day, bruised and laid across open windows, help to keep flies away from the house, but the herb is only effective while fresh and aromatic. For a spray against aphids, boil 220gr ($\frac{1}{2}$lb) tansy shoots in 1 litre of water for 10 minutes. Cool, thoroughly strain, add a couple of drops of washing up liquid and use within a day or so. Do not store.
CURLED TANSY *Tanacetum vulgare crispum* is a smaller growing cultivar (20–35cm) which, although it sends exploring rhizomes across any bed in which it is planted, has a pleasing 'Prince of Wales feather' form of leaf and the typical yellow button flowers.

TARRAGON, FRENCH
(Little Dragon)
Artemisia dracunculus
Perennial herb (40–50cm) dying down in winter. The fibrous roots send up tender shoots in late spring. It has linear grey-green leaves on branching stems and small flowers of ray florets, which are insignificant and sometimes absent.
Cultivation: French tarragon will flourish if its simple requirements are met. It prefers a rather poor soil in a well-drained, open and uncrowded situation. Grow at the front of a bed and, if the soil is at all heavy or inclined to get waterlogged in winter, plant the tarragon on top of a mound or ridge, like asparagus, so that surplus moisture can run from the roots. Incorporate some sandy compost in the soil before planting. French tarragon does not revert or become Russian tarragon, but it may fall victim to being given too rich a soil, too much watering and disturbance of the roots. When the plant dies down at the end of autumn, a little light sandy compost must be spread around it but care must be taken not to dig, fork or hoe close to the roots in spring or the tender underground shoots may be broken off before they have a chance to come through the soil. Propagation is by cuttings or division of roots in spring as French tarragon rarely sets viable seed. Any seed purchased as tarragon will almost certainly produce plants of

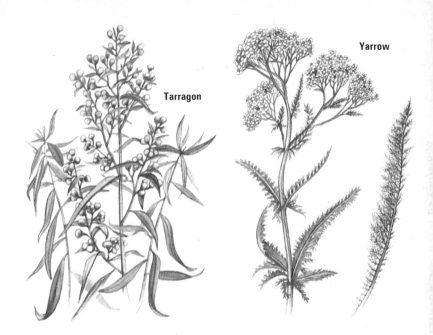

Tarragon

Yarrow

Russian tarragon *(Artemisia dracunculoides)* growing to 1m, with wider, lighter green leaves, often forked at the tips, and with little or no flavour.

Uses: the hot aromatic anise-like flavour of French tarragon is difficult to describe but most people agree that its piquancy contributes something quite special to chicken, turkey and pork dishes, gives a hot touch to a cool salad, and flavours vinegars, oils and jellies for use in various ways. Tarragon tea helps to banish indigestion.

YARROW

(Staunchweed, Soldiers Woundwort)
Achillea millefolium
A hardy perennial found growing wild on roadside verges, with creeping rootstock and finely cut leaves (5–10cm), each segment deeply indented giving a feathery effect. Basal leaves are stalked, those on the stems stalkless and shorter. Stems grow to 50–60cm and bear corymbs of dull white, pinkish or sometimes deep pink disc and ray florets, the flat heads 6–8cm across, which flower throughout the summer.

Cultivation: pieces pulled off at soil level, usually already rooted, will 'take' with no difficulty and spread rapidly.

Uses: the common names of this herb show that it was used as a styptic, a plant to stop bleeding. The generic name *Achillea* came from the legend that Achilles staunched the bleeding wounds of his soldiers with yarrow; the specific name *millefolium* describes the finely cut 'thousand leaves' of its growth. In less hygienic days than these a cobweb was placed over a wound to arrest the blood flow and help it to coagulate; the fine network of yarrow leaves might well achieve the same result. Taken in combination with elderflower and peppermint, fresh or dried, it is a favourite herbal infusion to be drunk at the first signs of a cold. A cool infusion of leaves used as a cosmetic wash is good for greasy skins, while the young basal leaves may be chopped into salads. Used as an activator, yarrow will help to break down garden rubbish for compost.

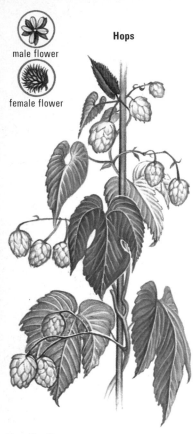

male flower

female flower

Hops

Family Cannabaceae

HOP
Humulus lupulus
Perennial with stout rootstocks which sends up tender shoots each year. These become tough twining stems (known as bines) which are capable of climbing to a considerable height. Male and female are different plants. The male produces loose panicles of tiny green flowers, while the female flowers are enclosed in round or oval papery yellow-green bracts known as strobiles (3–4cm in length). The rough textured leaves are heart-shaped and lobed with toothed edges, the upper leaves are smaller and sometimes without lobes.

Cultivation: from seed or suckers taken from strong female plants in spring. To produce good-sized hops the plant requires deeply-dug and well-manured soil. The plants can be trained as decorative climbers in a sunny airy position; the old bines should be cut out after the hops have matured to avoid tangled growth when the new shoots grow from the rootstocks the following spring. The commercial growing of hops in this country has always been confined to a few counties where the soil conditions are suitable, chiefly Kent, Herefordshire and Worcestershire. Precautions must be taken to prevent the spread of fungus diseases which endanger the crops; hops grown in gardens in these parts of the country should either be sprayed with a fungicide or watched very carefully for any sign of fungus or other infection and if detected the bines should be burnt at once.

Uses: Henry VIII forbade brewers to use the hop in ale, describing it as 'a wicked weed that would spoil the taste of the drink and endanger the people'. At that time it was thought to induce a state of melancholy. Herbs such as alecost, yarrow and wormwood were added to ale for their bitter or aromatic flavours, and the use of hops to give taste and to preserve the beverage was only later acquired from the Dutch and Germans and their name for it 'beer' adopted. A simple home brew can be made by putting 55gr (2oz) hops in 2.25 litres ($\frac{1}{2}$ gallon) boiling water for 15 minutes. Strain, then dissolve 0.45kg (1lb) brown sugar in the liquor. To this add 4.50 litres (1 gallon) of cold water and 2 tablespoonfuls of fresh yeast. Allow to stand for twelve hours and then bottle. Tea made from 2 or 3 hops and a teaspoonful of honey in a cupful of boiling water is a good tonic and sedative. Also hop leaves may be dried, crushed and added, half and half, to Ceylon or Indian teas. In spring tender young shoots, no more than 12cm high, can be picked, tied in bunches and cooked like asparagus. Small muslin bags stuffed with dried hops can be slipped into a pillowcase to help sufferers from insomnia, and in the past the khaki dyes needed for army uniforms were also made from hops.

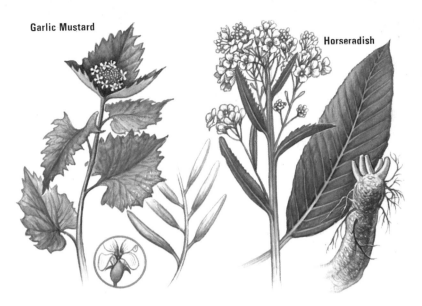

Garlic Mustard

Horseradish

Family Cruciferae

GARLIC MUSTARD
(Jack-by-the-hedge)
Alliaria petiolata
A biennial with an erect stem (30–90cm). The fresh green, stalked, heart-shaped leaves have toothed edges, and release a strong garlic smell when bruised. The small white flowers, which appear in spring, have 4 petals in cross formation and are arranged in a corymb. Garlic mustard can be found growing wild under hedgerows and in waste places.
Cultivation: by seed in late spring. The plant will self-sow when the seeds ripen late in the following spring or early summer and then die.
Uses: the young leaves used sparingly will give a garlic flavour to salads and other dishes and may be chopped into sauces (as the common name 'Sauce-alone' suggests). The plant has anti-septic properties and the juice is used to cleanse ulcers and skin eruptions. The leaves crushed until moist may be rubbed on to aching limbs to promote a feeling of warmth.

HORSERADISH
Armoracia rusticana
A hardy perennial herb cultivated by the ancient Egyptians and probably for centuries before their civilization. From the long tapering taproot (50–60cm) basal leaves grow to 50cm. Lanceolate with indented edges, and with a prominent midrib on the underside, the coarse leaves are often mistaken for docks. The flowering stems, bearing small leaves, terminate in small clusters of tiny 4-petalled white flowers.
Cultivation: pieces of root with a bud attached should be cut off in spring and planted in good deep soil. Horseradish spreads rapidly and must be kept to a part of the garden where it cannot become a nuisance. Every few years it is wise to dig up the old bed and replant.
Uses: best known as a sauce served with roast beef, but it is also good with fish. Home-made horseradish sauce is much hotter than that commercially produced. An infusion of a little scraped horseradish root with honey added may help to soothe a persistent cough; and a gentle massage with the cut root helps to warm stiff or aching joints.

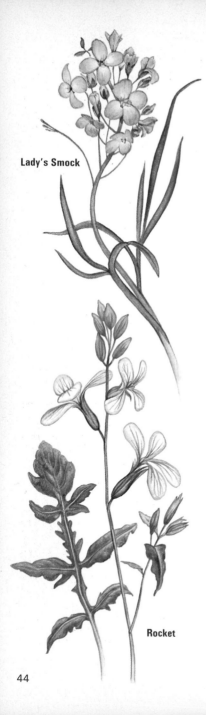

Lady's Smock

Rocket

LADY'S SMOCK
(Cuckoo flower)
Cardamine pratensis
This is one of the prettiest of spring wild flowers and welcome as a garden plant. Its name, cuckoo flower, associates it with the time the cuckoo returns to Britain, but the plant is widely distributed in northern Europe. It is a slender erect perennial (20–40cm) first showing a rosette of pinnate leaves with rounded leaflets. The stem leaflets which then appear are narrower; and the flowers, arranged in a raceme ($1\frac{1}{2}$–2cm), are 4-petalled and mauve-pink with darker mauve veining in the petals (occasionally double flowers occur).
Cultivation: from seed sown in spring. The plant does best in damp places and will grow in semi-shade.
Uses: like many so-called 'weeds' this plant has many virtues. It is rich in vitamin C and was a welcome blood-purifying herb in the spring when scurvy was an annual problem after winter months of food lacking necessary vitamins. Of the same family as watercress it makes a good substitute for it, as well as for mustard and cress. Good in salads and soups.

ROCKET
(Roquette)
Eruca versicaria subspecies *sativa*
An annual salad herb at first forming a rosette of dark green deeply-lobed leaves from which the purplish flower stem rises 20–50cm with narrower leaves and reddish flower buds opening to show 4 narrow petals with purple-brown veins (3cm).
Cultivation: it likes a moisture retaining soil in an open sunny position. Seed should be sown in succession from late spring to enable one to take tender young leaves from the quickly growing plants – the older leaves soon get coarse.
Uses: a salad herb with a cress flavour.
SWEET ROCKET *Hesperis matronalis* is a biennial producing a rosette of oblong leaves the first year, and a stem bearing heads of white or mauve sweetly scented flowers in the second year, before it dies. Grow where the scent will enable to waft in through open windows at night in summer.

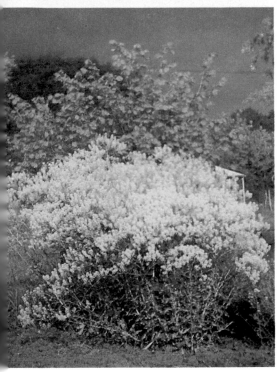

A colourful display of woad in flower in the author's garden. The blue dye so commonly used in the past comes from the leaves.

WOAD
(Dyer's woad)
Isatis tinctoria

Hardy biennial producing a rosette of oblong leaves in its first year, and then the second year sending up in early spring a tall, erect, branching stem (50–125cm), with small clasping leaves and terminal panicles of many small yellow 4-petalled flowers which make a fine show. As the plant matures the undersides of the leaves turn dark blue and this is where the colour for the dye comes from. The ripe brown-black seeds vary in size and hang for some considerable time in clusters which attract as much attention as the dense heads of tiny flowers.

Cultivation: from seed sown in late summer after it has ripened on the plant. It sometimes does not remain viable until the following spring.

Uses: people have been using the dye extracted from woad for around 2000 years. The ancient Britons dyed their bodies with it, using it as a warpaint to frighten their enemies. As it is a vulnerary it would also have helped to heal their wounds, but it should never be taken internally. Producing the dye from the plant was a complicated process. The leaves were ground to a pulp, then drained, rolled into balls and dried. After this they were ground to a powder which was piled on a stone floor in heaps and constantly sprinkled with water to cause it to ferment; this took many weeks until the mass became a dark clay-like substance, the dye. Apparently the smell during the fermenting process was obnoxious and it is said that Queen Elizabeth I commanded that no woad should be grown within several miles of her castles! It only ceased to be a commercial dye crop in the 1930s when synthetic dyes made growing it uneconomic.

Family Crassulaceae

HOUSELEEK
(Hen and Chickens)
Sempervivum tectorum
A perennial (to 8cm) forming a rosette of fleshy hairless leaves with prickles or spines at the tips. It does not flower regularly but when it does it sends up a scaly-leaved stem (15–25cm), with clusters of scentless pink flowers coming from one side only of the stem.
Cultivation: the tenacious fibrous roots will cling to dry rocky surfaces, walls and even roofs. The plant increases by young plantlets growing out from the side of the parent and spreads freely, so getting its name of hen and chickens.
Uses: when the leaf is sliced through horizontally the fleshy interior is cooling to the skin and may be applied to burns and inflamed areas; it has been used to treat warts and corns but should not be taken internally. Much superstition surrounds this plant. It has been grown on the roofs of houses since before the 1st century AD for it was thought to protect the inhabitants from fire, lightning and evil spirits. In fact the quickly-spreading plant may well have protected and helped to preserve thatched roofs. It makes a decorative plant for rockeries, troughs, walls or any extremely dry areas.

Family Chenopodiaceae

GOOD KING HENRY
(Mercury)
Chenopodium Bonus Henricus
A hardy perennial herb with taproots and stems (to 50cm) bearing dark green, stalked, arrow-shaped leaves, the undersides mealy to the touch. The flowers are dense spikes of tiny green blooms and as the seed ripens the spikes bend into the shape of a crook.
Cultivation: by seed sown in spring or late summer or by cutting old roots into pieces retaining a bud or growing point; this can be done in spring or autumn. The established plants will seed freely.
Uses: a rather unattractive looking plant but it is rich in iron and is a nutritious cut-and-come-again vegetable. When it is coming through in spring the young growth can be blanched by covering it with a pot or bucket – the tender pink shoots are good in early salads. Later, as the uncovered herb grows, the leaves should be picked frequently, and flower stems should be cut out as they appear, otherwise the leaves become small, coarse and bitter. If seeds are wanted, leave one plant to grow on, flower and ripen seed.

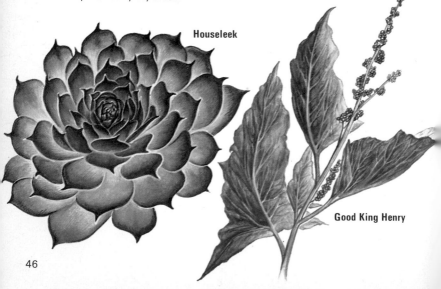

Houseleek

Good King Henry

FAT HEN

(Goosefoot, Lambs Quarters)
Chenopodium album
A prolific annual herb (to 75cm) found on roadside dumps and field verges. The erect branching stems bear grey-green leaves, oval or arrow-shaped, and mealy on the undersides. The insignificant green flowers grow in short dense spikes from midsummer.

Cultivation: by seed; it will grow in poor soil but given better conditions it makes stocky healthy plants.

Uses: this plant is rich in iron, calcium, vitamins B1 and C, and has been a valuable source of food since prehistoric times. It is a member of the same family as cultivated spinach, but more nutritious. Like Good King Henry, it should be cut frequently to produce a good growth of leaves. In the past the seed was ground and used as flour, and the plant gets its name of fat hen from being fed to poultry to fatten them. The young stalks are succulent and tender when cooked but they get rather tough when fully grown.

ORACH

(Arrach, Mountain spinach)
Atriplex hortensis
A hardy annual appearing in late spring. The branching stems (70–100cm) have stalked, opposite, arrow-shaped leaves with toothed edges, which feel mealy to the touch. The flowers are in red spikes, and the round flat seeds, encased in bracts, are red at first, changing to biscuit brown when ripe.

Cultivation: the plant grows easily from seed but it is best sown in the place it is to grow as it does not transplant well. It will respond to good soil and make much bushier plants than in poor soil.

Uses: Orach is notable for the rich beetroot colour of its stems and leaves and it can look very striking grown with grey and soft green foliage plants. The leaves are almost transparent and if it is planted where sunlight can shine through them it adds to its beauty. It may be cooked, like spinach, in very little water; the red colour comes out of the leaves leaving a green vegetable.

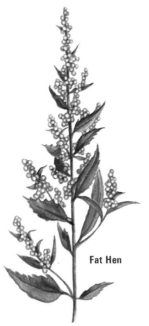

Fat Hen

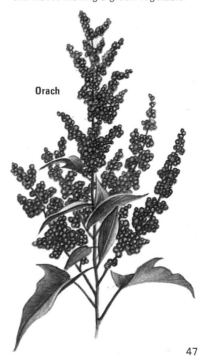

Orach

47

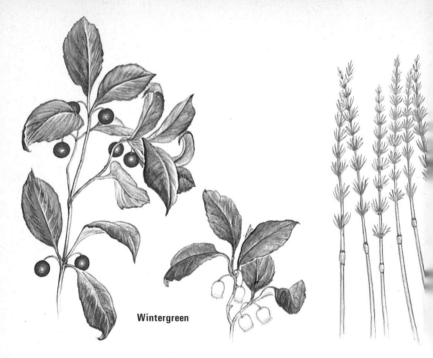

Wintergreen

Family Ericaceae

WINTERGREEN
(Mountain Tea)
Gaultheria procumbens
A native of North America, named after Dr Gaultier who practised medicine in Quebec in the mid 18th century. It is an evergreen perennial (to 15cm) with creeping stems which become woody. The oval leaves (1½–5cm) are dark green, shiny on the upper surfaces and paler beneath, with shallowly serrated edges. The white bell-shaped flowers (5–7mm) hang singly from the leaf bases and bloom from midsummer, maturing to red berries in autumn.

Cultivation: by cuttings or division of root in spring or seed (berries) in autumn. It is a member of the heather family and likes a lime-free peaty soil.

Uses: the leaves when bruised or broken give off a warm aromatic smell familiar to those who remember having their chest rubbed for coughs and colds. The oil is employed in a 'rub' used externally for rheumatic and muscular pains and to flavour dental preparations. A few leaves may be infused to make an aromatic tea. Wintergreen is a good ground cover plant for semi-shady areas or to grow between shrubs like rhododendrons or azaleas which need a lime-free soil. The genus includes many small, low-growing, spreading shrubs which may be cultivated for the interest of their foliage, flowers and berry fruits. The English Wintergreens, species of *Pyrola*, are not related.

Family Equisetaceae

HORSETAIL
(Pewterwort)
Equisetum arvense
The horsetails, of which there are several species, form a single genus *Equisetum*. They have survived since the carboniferous period, maintaining their strange habit of growth. Common horsetail is a perennial with creeping rhizomes. Early in spring fertile brown

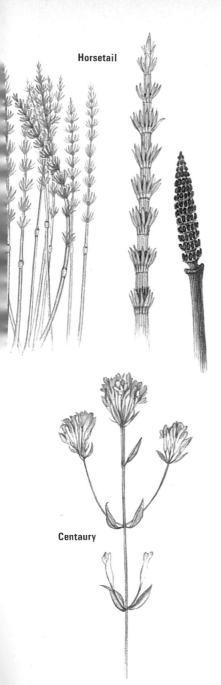

Horsetail

Centaury

shoots grow 14–20cm with terminal spore-bearing cones which shed their spores and then die. These are followed by green infertile stems (20–100cm), from the nodes of which grow whorls of segmented lateral branches.

Cultivation: short lengths of rhizome will root quickly in most soils and care must be taken to ensure that this herb does not become a noxious weed in the garden as it spreads at an alarming rate and is not easy to eradicate.

Uses: in the past, horsetail has been used as a poultice to be applied externally to wounds and ulcers; and taken as a tea for the treatment of bladder complaints. The stems contain silicic acid which helps the growth of healthy finger nails. The dried stems, rolled into a ball, can be used as a pan scourer and its common name of pewterwort was acquired because it was so successful for polishing this metal and also for cleaning woodwork.

Family Gentianaceae

CENTAURY
(Centre of the Sun)
Erythraea centaurium
An annual with yellowish fibrous roots and erect square stems (to 30cm). It has light green, oblong basal leaves and opposite, stalkless stem leaves which become narrower as they reach the terminal branching clusters of bright pink tubular flowers, coming into bloom at midsummer. The name centaury is thought to have come from the Centaur Chiron, famed in Greek mythology for his skill in the use of medicinal plants; attention was first drawn to the herb because of his claim that it had cured him of a wound from a poisoned arrow.

Cultivation: from seed sown in spring on the surface of the soil in a sunny well-drained position. The plants will self-sow but do not like being transplanted.

Uses: the herb is bitter to taste but it is a good simple tonic, will stimulate a reluctant appetite and helps the digestion. This is a delightful small herb which can be grown in a rockery or trough garden and will naturalize between paving or gravel.

49

Family Guttiferae

ST JOHN'S WORT
Hypericum perforatum
A stiff-stemmed perennial (50–60cm) with dense creeping rootstock. The light green leaves are oblong, linear and opposite, and there are terminal cymes of golden-yellow flowers which have 5 petals and many stamens. The leaves and petals are dotted with oil glands. In bloom towards the end of June for St John's Day, the plant was dedicated to the saint, but it was being used medicinally long before his time.

Cultivation and uses: may be grown from seed in spring or division of root in spring or autumn; it likes an open position and light soil. It yields a red oil used externally to treat aching joints, wounds and burns, which is thought to be antibiotic and antiviral.

Witch Hazel

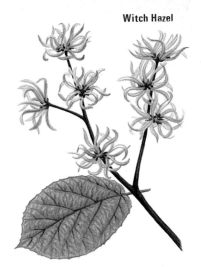

Family Hamamelidaceae

WITCH HAZEL
Hamamelis virginiana
A deciduous shrub (3–4m) with smooth, dull grey-green bark. The leaves (5–10cm) are oval to obovate, downy and roundly toothed. In autumn after the leaves have fallen, shaggy-petalled yellow flowers, brown inside, appear.

Cultivation and uses: this ornamental shrub needs a semi-shady position and a humus-rich soil. Mulching with leafmould will prevent the soil drying out, which can be fatal to this plant. (Always put mulch down on soil that is already moist; if it covers dry soil the rain may not be able to penetrate through it down to the roots). Witch hazel is a North American native shrub and it was the Indians who taught the early settlers of its healing properties. Distilled witch hazel is a soothing astringent for skin complaints and is used as an eye lotion and for insect bites. The Chinese witch hazel *(H. mollis)* is a large handsome shrub with fragrant flowers in bloom from December to March, a time when flowers of any kind are welcome.

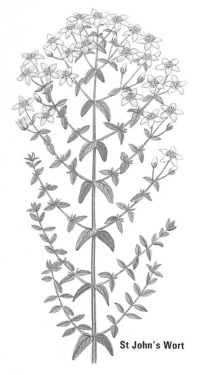

St John's Wort

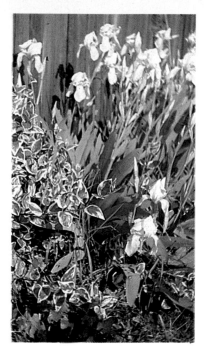

Orris is an early flowering, elegant iris. The violet-scented root is used in toilet preparations.

Family Iridaceae

ORRIS

Iris germanica var. *florentina*
A perennial (30–40cm) with thick rhizomes and sword-shaped leaves. The stems bear heads of white, purple-streaked flowers in late spring.

Cultivation: from rhizomes taken from the rootstock in spring or autumn and lightly pushed into the soil (do not bury them) in a well-drained open position.

Uses: a pleasing early-flowering iris to grow. Those interested in making pot pourri should detach some rhizomes, then peel, dry and grind them to use as a fixative to hold the scents and add a violet scent of its own. The dried orris must be stored in an airtight container; it may be a few weeks before the violet perfume can be detected.

SAFFRON
(Saffron Crocus)
Crocus sativus
A perennial similar in appearance to the spring-flowering crocus. The corm produces narrow grass-like leaves in late summer followed by purple flowers with prominent branching styles.

Cultivation: a good rich soil is required for the corm to produce flowers, and plants should be at least 10cm apart. The styles bearing the stigmas are the parts of the flower collected for drying and well over 4000 are needed to yield an ounce.

Uses: this scarce, highly-valued herb was greatly esteemed for its colour and perfume by the poets of ancient times. At one time it was grown commercially in England and the town of Saffron Walden testifies to the area having been well suited to its cultivation. Nowadays true saffron is used for colouring and flavouring rice, buns and cakes or can be taken as a tea for digestive troubles or as a light sedative. Care must be taken not to confuse saffron with the poisonous *Colchicum autumnale* (see page 121).

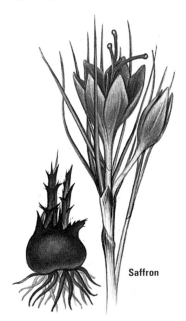

Saffron

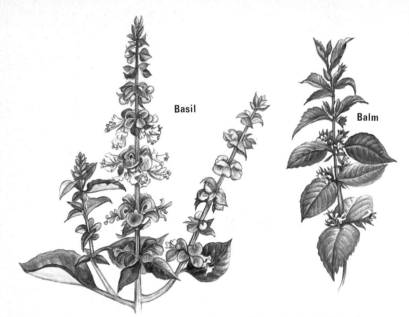

Basil

Balm

Family Labiateae

BASIL
(Sweet Basil)
Ocimum basilicum

A half-hardy annual with upright branching habit (30–40cm) and ovate shiny green leaves (3–5cm). The white-lipped flowers grow in whorls from the axils of the leaves, but are an insignificant part of the plant. When any part is bruised, the characteristic clove-like scent is evident. Bush basil *(Ocimum minimum)* grows as a smaller compact bush with leaves only 1½–2cm. Opal basil *(O. basilicum purpurascens)* has the habit of sweet basil, with beautiful purple leaves and a pink flower. Other members of the family include the sacred basil of India *(O. sanctum)* which the Indians call 'tulsi', the lettuce-leaved basil *(O. crispum)* and the lemon-scented lemon basil *(O. citriodorum)*.

Cultivation: all the basils are half-hardy in this country and the seed should not be sown out of doors before June. It can be sown indoors from late April but the young plants must not be planted out until mid-June, or when all danger of frosts and cold nights is over. In a good summer it will do well in a warm, well-drained, sheltered border, but it may be wise to keep some plants indoors if the weather is uncertain. Early autumn frosts will kill off outside plants but if a few are potted up and brought indoors they should go on into the winter.

Uses: basil is a herb of contradictions – its flavour is much sought after by many, but others find it quite unacceptable. In the past many legends have grown up around it. The Greeks thought it signified hatred and poverty and that it grew best when the seed was sown accompanied by curses and abuses, but in Italy it was given as a love token. In the past, some people believed that no foods could be eaten from a plate under which a sprig of basil had been placed, while others claimed that it 'procured a cheerful and merry heart'. Keats wrote a long poem about Isabella who buried her lover's head in a pot of basil; in Egypt women scattered basil on the graves of their loved ones. Today it is one of the most popular herbs in salads and pasta dishes, and is used with tomato in almost any context

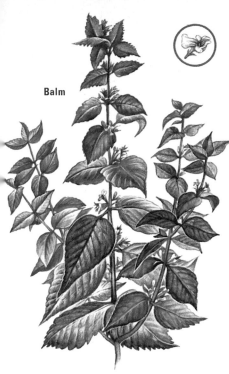

Balm

the leaves are bruised, makes it one of the favourite herbs to grow today, as it has been for thousands of years. Its name *Melissa* is derived from the Greek word for bee leaf; beekeepers used to grow the herb for the nectar it yields and rub it on their hives to attract swarms. The name 'balm' suggests its use as a mild sedative. An infusion made from the fresh leaves is a delicious summer drink, taken either hot or iced, which will act as a digestive after a meal. The fresh young leaves add a delicate lemon flavour to any dish and are good in salads, with fish, in banana sandwiches, and with other fruit. The leaves rolled into a ball to release the oil may be used to soothe stings and midge bites. The herb needs careful drying to preserve its scent and flavour and should be removed from its drying place as soon as it is crisp and then stored in an airtight container.

GOLDEN VARIEGATED BALM *(Melissa officinalis variegata)* is a radiant sight in spring when the leaves are bright golden. It loses its brilliant colour during the summer but is dappled with gold again in the autumn before dying down in winter.

The brilliant foliage of golden variegated balm is at its best in spring.

and as a herb to flavour oils and vinegars. The purple-leaved opal basil will please those interested in material for flower and foliage arrangements.

BALM
(Lemon Balm, Bee Balm)
Melissa officinalis
A hardy perennial growing into dense clumps (to 90cm). The square stems bear ovate leaves with crenate edges (5–8cm) growing in opposite pairs. The insignificant flowers, primrose-yellow in bud, open to white from midsummer.

Cultivation: by seed sown in spring or division of root in spring or autumn. Established plants self-sow freely, and the progress of balm through the garden will have to be controlled as young plants appear in unexpected places.

Uses: the refreshing lemon scent of this plant, although not evident before

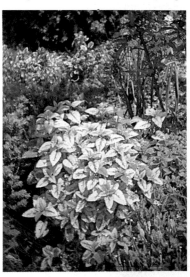

BERGAMOT
(Oswego Tea)
Monarda didyma and cvs
Herbaceous perennials dying down in winter and spreading out from the parent plants by rhizomes. The stems are square, erect (35–100cm) with slightly serrated ovate-lanceolate leaves in opposite pairs arranged alternately up the stem. The decorative whorled flowerheads show a random display of narrow, tubular florets with deeply cleft lips and visibly protruding stamens. There are crimson, scarlet, purple, lavender, pink and white bergamots but the most fragrant is *M. didyma*.

Cultivation: from seed sown in late spring or, to ensure true progeny from the parent plant, from rhizomes pulled from the outside of the plant in spring or early autumn. Bergamot is closely allied to the mints and likes the same conditions: a moist humus-rich soil with some shade during the hottest part of the day. After about three years the plants should be lifted, the original heart of the plant discarded and the healthy outside growth split into new clumps and replanted; if this is not done the plant loses its vigour and is inclined to die out. Young growth should be protected from slugs.

Uses: *M. didyma* has a delicious scent similar to the bergamot orange *(Citrus bergamia)* from which it gets its name and which yields the bergamot oil used in commerce. The lavender-coloured *M. fistulosum*, abundantly wild in North America where it is a native, is the Oswego Tea commonly drunk by the American Indians which became famous when it was adopted as a beverage by many Americans after the Boston tea party to demonstrate their protest against the tax imposed on imported tea. The white-flowered bergamot 'Snow Maiden' is not as common or robust as the other cultivars but its purity of colour and refreshing lemon scent are worth seeking. The early-flowering 'Croftway Pink' is thyme scented. Young bergamot leaves may be used in salads and fresh or dried for tisanes. It is interesting to note the subtle changes of flavour that are evolved by blending the leaves with 'ordinary' tea. Bergamot holds its scent well when carefully dried and is a valuable ingredient for pot pourri.

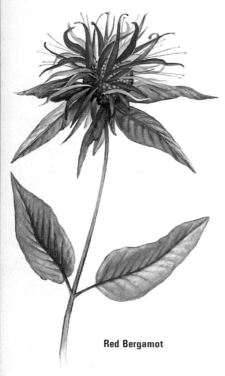

Red Bergamot

BETONY
(Wood Betony)
Stachys officinalis (Betonica offic.)
Perennial herb with some basal growth persisting through the winter. It has fibrous roots and the stems grow from a rosette of stalked leaves (to 30–50cm). The stem leaves, slightly hairy, are oval with crenate edges. The rosy-purple flowers appear first in whorls coming from the axils of the leaves and then as a dense terminal spike.

Cultivation: can be grown from seed sown in spring or late summer, or from rooted plantlets eased out of the parent plant in spring. It prefers a semi-shady position and is a pleasing-looking herb

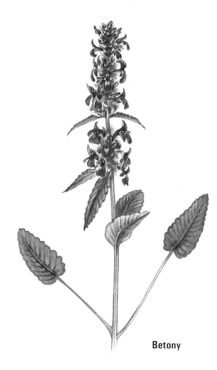

Betony

ground level, and oval and stalkless on the stems, which terminate in a spike formed by several whorls of flowers. These are blue-lipped with purple-blue bracts between the whorls, giving the whole a densely packed appearance.

Cultivation: the stolons root freely and it is possible to detach pieces with plantlets already formed at the nodes. Each plantlet will throw out rooting stems, so this herb makes an excellent ground cover plant where speed of growth is welcome. There are cultivars with bronze and cream and pink and green foliage which continue to show colour in winter.

Uses: the herb is bitter and astringent and for many centuries has had a reputation as a styptic and wound herb; its common names of sicklewort and carpenter's herb indicate its use in stopping the bleeding of cuts caused by accidents with tools.

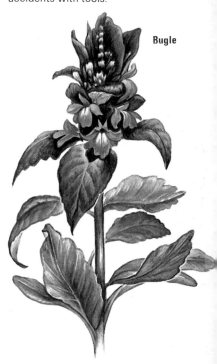

Bugle

with its rosette of shapely leaves in spring and spikes of flowers in summer.
Uses: quite extravagant claims have been made in the past for the medicinal and magical powers of betony. An infusion made from the herb will in fact act as a mild sedative to quieten anxiety or soothe headaches, and it is also useful as a good bitter tonic drink and, externally, for cleansing and helping to heal wounds. The dried leaves can be included in herbal smoking mixtures and are an ingredient of some snuffs. As a member of the woundwort family it is reasonable to use this herb to bathe sore places.

BUGLE
(Sicklewort, Carpenter's Herb)
Ajuga reptans
A perennial herb with spreading stolons sending up erect stems (10–15cm). It has opposite pairs of leaves which are oblong and stalked at

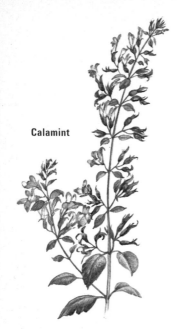

Calamint

CALAMINT
(Common Calamint)
Calamintha ascendens
A small branching hairy perennial (30–40cm) with oval leaves (2–3cm) with slightly serrated edges in opposite pairs. The flower stalks come from the axils of the leaves and form tapering spikes of pink-purple, narrow, tubular, lipped florets growing in clusters. The whole plant is warmly aromatic with a pepperminty taste and smell. It forms a neat bushy little plant.

Cultivation: from seed, cuttings or division of the root in spring. It likes a sunny well-drained position and fairly light soil and in these conditions it will seed itself. Cut the stems right down to the basal leaves after it has finished flowering unless ripe seed is needed.

Uses: a good digestive tea may be made from this herb, or it can be taken as a warming bedtime drink or to soothe a cough. It is worth drying some for winter use. Calamint is restrained in its growth and would do well on a rockery or in sink or trough gardens.

CATMINT
Nepeta faassenii (Nepeta mussini)
A hardy perennial dying down in the winter. In spring it sends up softly hairy grey-green serrated leaves (2–3cm) which form clumps of dense bushy growth 25–30cm tall and 50–60cm across. The flowers grow on long arching spikes and are a soft misty lavender blue.

Cultivation: catmint can be grown from seed sown in spring or division of root clumps in spring or autumn. It likes a well-drained soil and sunny position, and will come into flower in late spring. When the flower stalks have died off they should be removed, and the bush trimmed into a neat shape so that the foliage will give pleasure until it sends up a second crop of flowering stems. In late autumn about half the length of flowering stalks should be cut back, leaving some to give protection during the winter to the rootstock which is susceptible to damage from hard frosts and cold east winds. This protection will be increased if the plants are surrounded with a dressing of compost, leaf mould or peat. In spring, when the young shoots can be seen to be growing, the rest of the old growth should be removed. Your cat, or indeed any others in the neighbourhood, will find it a most desirable place in which to curl up on sunny days, to the detriment of the shape of the bushes; there seems to be no way of discouraging the feline fondness for catmint.

Uses: this is a favourite border plant because it makes a good low hedge and gives much the same misty blue effect as lavender. It has a strange scent, which is difficult to describe and not to everyone's taste, but as a decorative herb it has much to commend it. Catmint associates well with pinks and greys but is best kept apart from the bright blue of hyssop as the two shades seem to cancel each other out. Nepeta Six Hills Giant grows to a bigger bush (60cm) and has longer flower spikes, and Nepeta Souvenir d'André Chaudron has large flowers of deep blue-purple. This cultivar is not as hardy as the type but if it can be obtained is well worth cherishing.

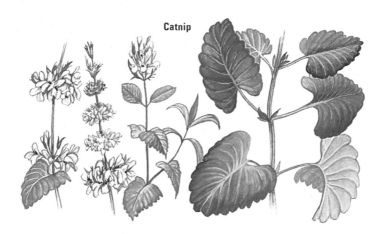

Catnip

CATNIP
(Catnep)
Nepeta cataria

This plant is best treated as a biennial as it has a habit of dying during the winter after flowering, particularly on heavier soils. It has not the attractive appearance of catmit, looking more like nettle or balm and growing upright (to 90–100cm). The ovate leaves have crenate edges and are in opposite pairs and in their axils whorls of small white-lipped flowers with purple dots appear.

Cultivation: on a light soil catnip grows easily from seed sown in spring or will self-sow from ripe seed in late summer. It is irresistibly attractive to cats and will need to be protected from them. There is an old saying:

'If you set it the cats will eat it,
'If you sow it the cat's won't know it.'

– in other words the sowing of seeds gives no smell of the herb but if it is handled for planting and the leaves or stems are bruised and release the smell, cats seem to come from miles around and will roll on it, eat it and in the end destroy it. If one is fond of cats this is definitely their herb and the dried leaves can be stuffed into pseudo 'mice' as playthings for them.

Uses: this is the medicinal catnip and the fresh or dried herb is used as an infusion for many minor complaints such as headaches, indigestion, colds, colic and diarrhoea. It may have a useful function in the garden as a spray against plant pests, using at least 55gr (2oz) fresh herb to 0.55 litre (1 pint) of water. Legend has it that chewing the root of catnip makes timid people brave and there is an account of a reluctant hangman who used to eat it to help him carry out his gruesome task.

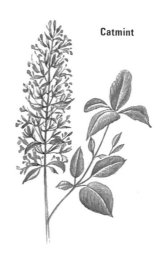

Catmint

GIPSYWORT
(Common Gipsyweed)
Lycopus europaeus
A perennial spreading by rhizomes and dying down in the winter. The erect stems (30–90cm) bear opposite pairs of lanceolate, sharply-toothed leaves (5–7cm). Dense whorls of mauve-spotted white-lipped flowers grow in the leaf axils from midsummer. A widely distributed herb found in damp places by lakes, riversides and canals.

Cultivation: will grow readily from pieces of rhizome pulled off the parent plant in spring or autumn and in damp situations it will spread rapidly. It is an interesting-looking plant with its sharply-pointed and indented leaves, the pairs arranged alternately forming a symmetrical pattern.

Uses: its names of gipsyweed or Egyptian's herb connect it with those nomads who find temporary stopping places near water. The herb yields a black dye used over thousands of years for dyeing fabrics and it was probably also used by the gipsies to keep their hair the dark colour so characteristic of their race. In the past gipsywort has been used in medicine in various ways. An infusion, though bitter to the taste, is useful as a sedative.

GROUND IVY
(Alehoof, Lizzy-run-up-the-hedge, Gill-run-over-the-ground)
Glechoma hederacea
A creeping perennial rapidly covering the ground and climbing into adjacent shrubs and bushes. The probing stems and the many opposite kidney-shaped leaves with crenate edges are softly hairy. The lipped flowers are lilac-coloured and persist from late spring to midsummer.

Cultivation: where natural ground cover is needed in a shady, rather damp place, ground ivy will soon provide it, but care must be taken not to let it invade any area of the garden where it may become a nuisance as the stems running over the ground root at their nodes and it spreads very quickly.

Uses: this herb has been used for many thousands of years to bathe sore eyes and bruises; and Gill tea was a popular spring tonic drink and digestive. Ground ivy is a bitter herb and the infusion is made more palatable if it is sweetened with honey. Its common name 'alehoof' reflects the fact that it was considered of value in brewing before hops were used; it was thought not only to flavour and preserve the ale but to help it to clear, and for this reason was used in the making of other drinks. Dried and finely powdered it became a snuff herb.

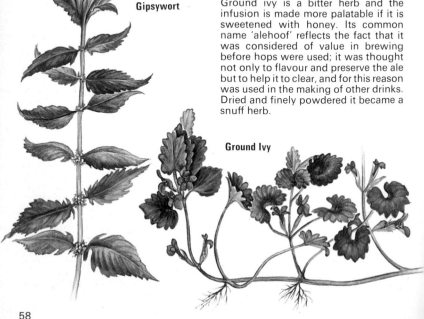

Gipsywort

Ground Ivy

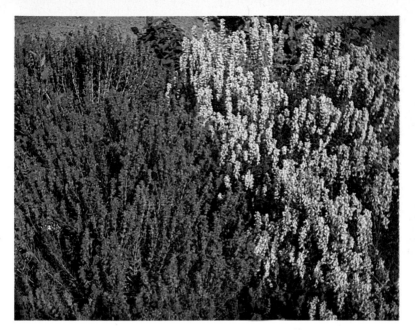

HYSSOP
Hyssopus officinalis

A woody perennial herb making a bush 60cm tall and 50cm across when in flower. The stems are branched and the linear, entire leaves (1½–3cm) are stalkless. The bright gentian-blue lipped flowers grow in whorls from one side of the stem forming a spike.

Cultivation: hyssop can be grown from seed sown in spring or early autumn. Pink hyssop *(H. officinalis rosea)* and white hyssop *(H. officinalis alba)* may also be grown from seed but their progeny may revert back to the blue type. To ensure that the pink, white or blue colours are reproduced, propagation should be from cuttings, best taken in spring. Hyssop does well in most soils but likes a sunny position and after flowering it should be cut back to a good shape. It responds well to this trimming which prevents it becoming too woody and tending to break away from the centre of the bush. The blue, pink or white hyssops make good low hedges and if kept regularly trimmed will last for many years; they become a mass of flower spikes giving a

Blue and white hyssop bushes, massed with densely packed flower spikes

wonderful show of colour, rather like large heathers. The pink and white merge well with catmint, lavender or grey foliage plants; the rich blue keeps its colour well and does not fade. Hyssops attract butterflies, an added bonus of colour. There is a dwarf cultivar, the blue rock hyssop *(H. aristatus)* of compact growth, about half the size of the type.

Uses: there have been differences of opinion as to whether the hyssop mentioned in the Bible was *Hyssopus officinalis* or one of the marjorams or the caper plant. Hyssop has a clean, wholesome smell reminiscent of cough medicines and a tea made from it can be soothing for a troublesome cough. The oil from the flowers and leaves has antiseptic properties and may help to soothe bruises and aching joints. It has also been used in perfumery and liqueurs. Hyssop helps to stimulate the appetite and tender young leaves can be added to salads or soups.

59

LAVENDERS

One of the best known and loved of all the herbs, grown in many gardens where no special thought has been given to herbs as such. *Lavandula vera* ('true'), *L. spica* ('spike') and *L. officinalis* ('the official one') have evolved as two main types – *L. angustifolia* (narrow-leaved) and *L. latifolia* (broad-leaved) – but there are many hybrids and cultivars.

Cultivation: all lavenders are bushy perennials and most are hardy. Originally from warm Mediterranean countries, they like as sunny a position as possible and if the garden is exposed to east wind they will appreciate some shelter. The soil should be well drained and compost or manure dug in at planting, and then as a mulch in autumn, to encourage good growth and flower production. If the soil is deficient in lime, a dressing should be given in spring. The bushes should be kept trimly in shape and all dead flowering stalks removed in autumn; if there is a heavy snowfall in winter, tap the bushes lightly with a stick to knock off the snow, otherwise its weight may split the bushes. Lavender grown from seed may not come true, so it is best to take cuttings. Short side shoots about 8cm are pulled off with a heel and all but the terminal leaves removed; the cuttings can be started in pots, boxes or the open ground if given some protection from strong sunlight. Plant firmly and during the winter check cuttings out of doors in case frosts have loosened the soil around them, exposing young roots.

Uses: lavender for drying should be cut when about half the blooms on the spike are expanded otherwise some may discolour or drop before all are in bloom. It is easier to rub the dried blooms off the stalks if all the flowerheads are kept facing one way. A small posy of lavender spikes pressed now and then to release the oil is an effective insect repellent. The florets can be used in salads and tisane made from lavender, fresh or dried, is a pleasant mild sedative. Lavender oil has many commercial uses in perfumery. Lavender bushes fall into three groups, large, semi-dwarf and dwarf.

OLD ENGLISH
Lavandula angustifolia

Large (90cm high, 80–100cm across when in flower). Narrow grey-green leaves and flowering stems (30–45cm) with tapering spike (8cm) of pale lavender colour. Blooms end of July to August and has a faintly camphor-like scent, but is not the best variety to grow for well-scented dried lavender. Its late flowering allows a succession of blooming if grown with other varieties.

DUTCH or GREY HEDGE
L. latifolia

The same habit and flowering time as Old English but the leaves are broader and a more silvery grey. The foliage of this lavender looks well in winter and compensates for the rather sparse display of long, pointed flowers, which are pale-coloured like Old English.

MUNSTEAD
L. angustifolia

Semi-dwarf (75cm high and 55–75cm across when in flower). This cultivar, which has proved to be one of the finest lavenders, owes its name to one of the most famous gardeners of all time, Gertrude Jekyll, who bred it at her Munstead Wood garden. The bush grows in compact form with bunches of dull grey, incurved leaves coming from the branched stems. The flower stalks terminate in a blunt-tipped spike of dark purple-blue florets of good perfume. Munstead is one of the earliest lavenders to bloom in July and if the first spikes are cut for drying or removed when the flowers are over, others will follow, extending the period of blooming for some weeks. If planted as a low hedge, for which it is unrivalled, the plants should be set 75cm apart.

PINK
L. rosea

Similar to Munstead in size and habit. The flower spikes look white until the florets open and show their pink colour. The short blunt heads (3–5cm) are sweetly scented. This lavender may look a little pallid on its own but complements the deep colours of Munstead or Hidcote.

HIDCOTE BLUE
L. nana atropurpurea
Dwarf (50cm high and 40–50cm across when in flower). The magnificent gardens of Hidcote Manor produced this lavender, which has the darkest blue colour of all the varieties. It grows as a neat bush and makes a very effective edging plant because of its incomparable colour, although the scent is not good. Set plants 45cm apart. There is also a cultivar, Hidcote Purple.

WHITE
L. nana alba
A choice little lavender of neat habit with short, blunt, well-scented flower-heads (2–3cm). It is not quite as hardy as the other lavenders and should be given a protected site with good drainage. Mulch with compost before winter to give protection through the bad weather.

FRENCH
L. stoechas
This sprawling Mediterranean species is not fully hardy in cold parts of the country. It should be given a very sheltered position and may be best kept in the greenhouse or a cool room in the house in winter. The interesting part of the plant is its purple flower spike surmounted by purple bracts which look rather like wings or a bow. Similar are Spanish lavender *(L. pedunculata)* with longer terminal dark purple bracts and *L. dentata* with deeply-toothed silver grey foliage.

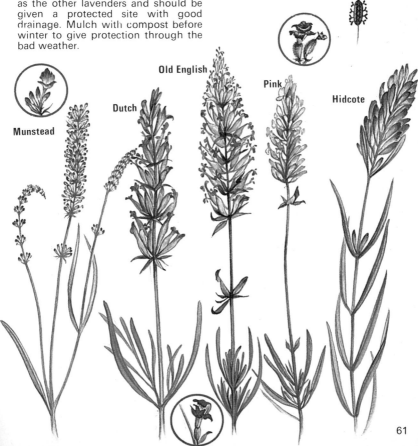

Munstead

Dutch

Old English

Pink

Hidcote

SWEET MARJORAM
(Knotted Marjoram)
Origanum marjorana

In warm climates this herb can be classed as a perennial but in Britain it is best treated as a half-hardy annual as it does not survive cold conditions out of doors. Growing on fibrous roots it forms an erect branching plant (20–30cm), with elliptical grey green opposite leaves (to 3cm) and spherical flower buds looking like tight knots, from which it gets its name 'knotted marjoram'. The insignificant small white flowers arranged in a corymb are in little clusters. The noteworthy feature of this marjoram is its delicious warm aromatic fragrance which prompted one of the herbalists of old to say that it 'should be given to those suffering from overmuch sighing'. Its scent is so good it *must* have a cheering effect!

Cultivation: from seed sown indoors in late April or May, or outside in June when all danger of frost is past. It needs a well-drained light soil and a sunny sheltered position with no overcrowding. The other members of the marjoram family are hardy, trouble-free perennials, but despite the somewhat tender nature of this plant every effort should be made to grow it, as it has one of the most pleasing fragrances of all the herbs. If some plants are lifted from the garden and potted up at the end of the summer and are brought indoors for protection before the frost can catch them, sweet marjoram will survive to give a welcome reminder of summer when the weather is cold and dull in November and December.

Uses: this lovely little herb can be made into a refreshing fragrant tea which is also good as an aid to digestion or as a mild expectorant for coughs. It is good with salads, tomato or egg dishes, in pizzas and freshly chopped as a garnish for cream soups, courgettes and avocado dishes. Like many herbs it is best added to cooked dishes just before serving as overcooking spoils its flavour. The dried herb is an excellent ingredient for pot pourri or to hang in muslin bags under the hot water tap of the bath. When travelling in hot weather take a few sprigs for its refreshing scent.

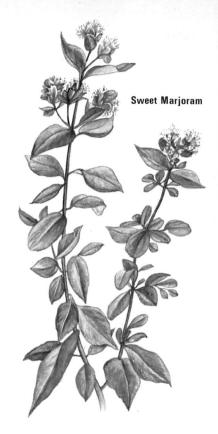

Sweet Marjoram

OREGANO
(Wild Marjoram, Origano)
Origanum vulgare

A compact low growing perennial with fibrous roots. The densely growing erect stems, sometimes reddish, make a bushy plant (to 45cm) and, like the pointed ovate dark green leaves (2–3cm), are hairy. The small pinkish-purple flowers are arranged in corymbs and bloom from midsummer to autumn. Wild marjoram is found on warm sunny banks, cliff-tops and rocky areas in limestone districts.

Cultivation: it can be grown from seed but as the marjorams are apt to hybridize it is wise to start with plants of the true *Origanum vulgare*. At certain times of the year the different marjorams can look much alike but they each have characteristic scents and if one can get to know these, identification is made easier. The aroma of oregano is sweet, round and warm. Established plants can be split into small clumps in spring and replanted in quite poor soil (similar to the conditions in which they would be found when growing wild); the less lush the plant grows the more intense is the flavour. Heavy soils can be made lighter by the addition of sandy compost, leaf mould and peat. Most aromatic plants appreciate lime and a dressing can be given in spring but, unless the soil is very heavy and sticky, once every three years will be sufficient.

Uses: a pleasant tea is made from oregano which will settle a disturbed stomach or help to ease a headache. The herb is used in many meat dishes, with pizzas, pastas, salads and soups, and associates well with mushrooms.

POT MARJORAM
Origanum onites

A hardy easily-grown perennial with a bushy habit. The erect stems bear opposite, light green, pointed ovate leaves (3–5cm) and the herb makes a clump 50cm high and 60cm across. The corymbs of flowers are mauve-pink or sometimes white. The scent of pot marjoram is sharper and less sweet than that of oregano.

Cultivation: from seed or division of the clumps in spring. Given an open sunny position pot marjoram will flourish on most soils and self-seed freely. If marjoram is to be dried for winter use, the herb should be cut as it is coming into flower in early summer; this trimming back will stimulate new growth and the bushes will send up new flowering stalks so that it is often possible to take three cuttings from the plants during the growing season. In late autumn if there are dead flowering stems left they should be cut off and the bushes trimmed back to a neat round shape.

Uses: the word 'pot' before this marjoram is an abbreviation of 'pottage' meaning a soup or stew or dish of lentils or pulses. The herb earned its prefix because it was so commonly added to these, but it is also used to flavour meat, fish, egg and cheese dishes, as well as sauces and salads. Marjoram tea has been a simple medicinal aid for hundreds of years in the treatment of nervous headaches and nausea, and long ago was recommended for seasickness, to prevent 'the wamblings of the stomach'. The oils in many of the herbs are antiseptic and cleansing and the various marjorams were used, like lemon balm, to rub down and clean wooden furniture and impart a wholesome fragrance to the air. Washing in water steeped in the herb has a beneficial effect on the skin.

One of the easiest and hardiest herbs to grow, pot marjoram has many uses in cooking and simple medicinal remedies.

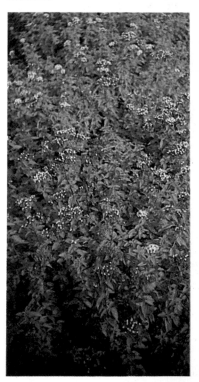

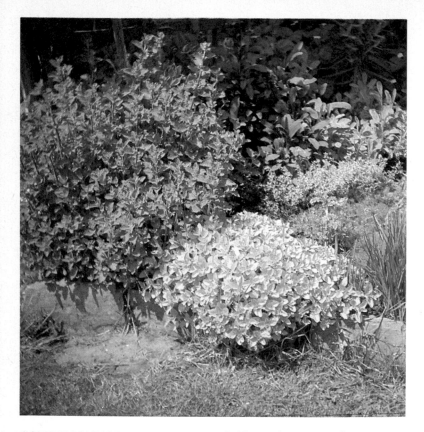

GOLDEN MARJORAM
Origanum aureum
A hardy perennial with a semi-procumbent habit. The persistent rootstock sends up hairy stems (35cm) with a dense growth of opposite and alternate golden-green, ovate leaves (2cm) and corymbs of pink or sometimes white flowers in tight clusters. The foliage has a pleasant lavender-like perfume when bruised.
Cultivation: can be grown from seed or root division. As with all the perennial marjorams it is usually easy to find many rooted pieces at ground level at the base of the herb and these, set into a sandy compost or light soil, will soon grow. Given a sunny position this

Golden marjoram grows into compact, cushion-like fragrant plants.

marjoram will make a cushion of golden foliage throughout the summer. If the dead top growth is trimmed off at the end of autumn, the basal leaf growth continues to give golden colour in the winter. Golden marjoram is a good subject for rockeries, to hang over steps or walls or to grow in gaps between paving. On light soil it will self-sow.
Uses: the lavender scent of this marjoram makes it useful for drying for pot pourri and sweet herb bath bags. It can be used in salads and makes a very pleasant tisane.

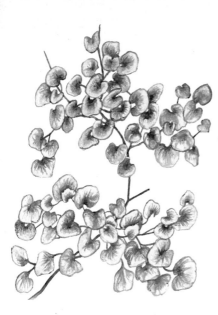

Curled Golden Marjoram

GOLDEN TIPPED MARJORAM
Origanum vulgare variegatum
This cultivar grows in exactly the same way as oregano, but in spring and early summer the dark green leaves are a bright golden colour for a third of their length to the tips. This interesting marking distinguishes the herb from its wild parent. In the summer the golden tip disappears and the bush looks just like, and can be used as, oregano; in the autumn some colour returns for a brief period and during the winter the leaves are green.
Cultivation: the same as for oregano. This herb is hardy and easy to grow and should be propagated vegetatively, by cuttings or division of root to ensure that the golden-tipped characteristic is passed on to the new plant.
Uses: for culinary and medicinal purposes it can be used as oregano but while it is displaying its colour marking it will be an interesting feature in the herb bed.

CURLED GOLDEN MARJORAM
Origanum aureum crispum
A neatly-growing small herb with fibrous roots. The stems are erect (to 25cm) with kidney-shaped crinkle-edged leaves that are bright gold during the summer. As the strength of the sun decreases, the leaves tend to become less golden and in the winter they are green. The small clusters of flowers may be pink or white.
Cultivation: this marjoram responds to a sunny position, as do other members of the family, but as it is less robust than other perennial relatives it should be given light soil, or heavy soil made light for its benefit. It is a charming little plant and one of the smaller herbs suitable for a trough garden.
Uses: it can be eaten or used for a tea but its interesting crinkly golden foliage is so attractive it is a pity to cut it off.

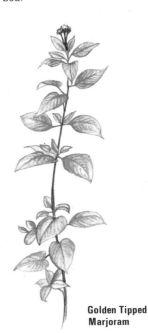

Golden Tipped Marjoram

MINTS

The genus Mentha is one of the most interesting groups of herbs, differing in size, habit, marking, colour and smell to such an extent that it may be difficult to believe that they all belong to the same family. Indeed it has been said that the mints pose more problems of identification and classification than any other genus of comparable size. Anyone who has grown mint over a number of years may have noticed that plants which could once be turned into a delicious mint sauce somehow lose their flavour, become rank and may no longer look exactly the same as when first planted. A mint bed grows vigorously at first and then has a tendency to become an overgrown tangle of roots all competing for nourishment. It is a greedy plant and to do well needs a rich moisture-retaining soil. Because it grows so fast when first planted, taking advantage of all available nourishment in the soil, do not feed it if you want to restrict its growth and stop it spreading. It may be put in a bottomless bucket or have tiles sunk around it to restrain it, but it will still escape or, if it exhausts the soil and becomes too dry, it will start to deteriorate. The plant grows and spreads by rhizomes, shallowly rooting stems which probe out in all directions for food. If it is to be kept growing healthily in one place, all the old growth should be dug and discarded at least every three years, and the ground replanted with strong young rhizomes taken from the outside of the parent plants. Dig some good compost into the soil at the same time. If the variegated-leaved cultivars are grown for their colour effect in herb beds, one has to be ruthless in carrying out the same procedure, otherwise the rhizomes will creep through the bed, coming up in the middle of other subjects and defeating the object of the original planting scheme. Most of the mints have evolved from the native cornmint *(M. arvensis)*, water mint *(M. aquatica)*, apple mint *(M. suaveolens)* and the naturalized spearmint *(M. spicata)*. From these parents have come innumerable hybrids and back to them many mints to some degree revert. If a survey was taken of the mint grown in gardens throughout the country for mint sauce the variety of hybrids found would be enormous.

Cultivation: all mints are perennials. It is difficult to ensure that those grown from seed will come true and to be certain of this they should be propagated by division of rhizomes in spring and autumn, planting into a good moisture-retaining soil. If any sign of deterioration or reversion is detected the roots should be dug up and burnt. In some seasons mints are affected by a fungus disease (rust), small brown spots appearing first on the undersides of the leaves and then quickly spreading. The condition does not get better but rapidly infects all the mint, so all affected growth should be cut off and burnt immediately.

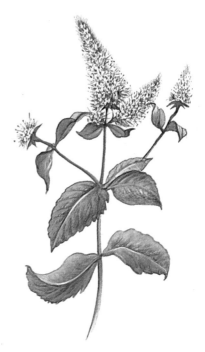

Apple Mint

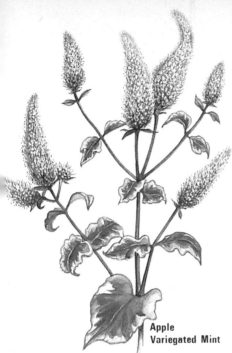

**Apple
Variegated Mint**

APPLE VARIEGATED MINT
M. suaveolens variegata
Growing to 60cm it has prettily marked leaves with white edges or white blotches on the outsides of the leaves. Sometimes entirely white shoots appear. It is a decorative plant for the garden and as a pot plant drapes well over the edges of the pot. The scent is good and it can be used for cooking, mint tea or dried for sweet bags or pot pourri. Always propagate from runners which are producing well-marked foliage.

BUDDLEIA MINT
M. longifolia
The robust mint (50–75cm) has pointed smoothly hairy leaves (6–9cm) with a camphoraceous smell. The flowers are in long pointed spikes of mauve whorled florets like the flower spikes of the buddleia shrub from which it gets its common name. The flavour is not good for sauce, but a tea made from it will make a soothing drink for coughs and colds.

APPLE MINT and BOWLES MINT
Mentha suaveolens and *M suaveolens rotundifolia* var. *Bowles*
These are two very similar species and are sometimes confused as the Bowles mint is often listed as 'Apple' mint. Their erect stems (to 90cm) have hairy, grey-green leaves which are both opposite and alternate. The flowers are in dense whorls forming a rather blunt spike. The leaves of Bowles mint are round, to 7cm long and 4cm broad. Both these mints have a good flavour with a fresh apple undertone. Bowles mint is very hardy, sometimes surviving a mild winter without dying back, and is more rust resistant than other mints. For sauce, mint jelly or tea either of these mints are excellent and one should not be discouraged from using them because of the hairy appearance of the leaves. The flavour of all mints gets stronger and sometimes rank in a dry season, when the plant is in flower. If it is cut back tender new growth will soon appear.

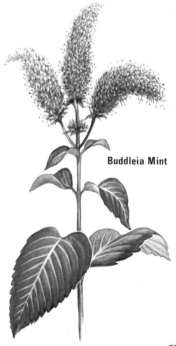

Buddleia Mint

EAU DE COLOGNE MINT
(Orange Mint)
M. x piperita cv. citrata

A strong-growing mint with branching erect stems (to 60cm) and bronze-green ovate leaves (5cm). The mauve flowers are in dense rounded terminal clusters, blooming from midsummer. This delightfully perfumed herb is one of the most popular mints for drying for pot pourri and sweet herb bags or to have in open bowls in a room. It may help to discourage flies and a fresh bunch carried in the car on a long journey can be wonderfully refreshing. This mint can be used as a garnish with fresh fruit or to float in fruit drinks, but it lacks the sharpness of spearmint or applemint and is too scented to make good mint sauce.

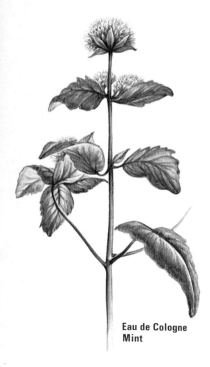

Eau de Cologne Mint

PINEAPPLE MINT
M. citrata cv.

A handsome mint growing with a rather spreading habit and much-branched stems (30–50cm). The striking yellow and green striped leaves are ovate and shiny, with a fragrance which, if not exactly like pineapple, is certainly fruity. The rhizomes branch freely and are noticeably whiter than some of the other mints. If it is ruthlessly kept within bounds this is a colourful mint, particularly in spring before the plant develops flowering shoots with their short round heads. It can be employed as a ground cover plant where its spreading habit is welcome. After flowering, towards the end of summer, if it looks a bit tatty, cut off the ragged growth and it will grow again, looking attractive until it dies down for the winter.

GINGER MINT
M. gentilis

Often confused with variegated apple mint as they both have the same slightly hairy texture and dull surface to the leaves. Whereas variegated apple mint has distinctive white edging to the leaves, ginger mint, although variable in its marking (sometimes having wholly green leaves, sometimes ones with random cream blotches) has an interesting, clearly defined half-and-half colouring displayed on some leaves, one side of the central vein being green and the other side cream. The cream and green marking becomes more evident as the plant matures. The terminal leaf buds are also a creamy colour, rather than the white of variegated apple mint. When crushed the leaves have a gingery smell and this becomes a pleasant fragrance when the herb is dried for adding to pot pourri. Ginger mint is also used as a herb tea.

LEMON MINT
(Bergamot mint)
M. aquatica cv. citrata

This mint grows to 50cm with branching stems and dull green, ovate leaves, sometimes showing a reddish flush on their undersides (to 4cm). Purple flowerheads appear as whorls in leaf axils and rounded terminal clusters, from midsummer. The scent of lemon mint is a delightful surprise from a rather unprepossessing-looking plant: a combination of lemon, bergamot and mint which is exhilarating. It makes a pleasant tea and for a mint sauce with special interest, use this mint with lemon juice instead of vinegar.

SPEARMINT
(Pea mint, Fish mint)
M. spicata (M. viridis)
A common garden mint (50–70cm) with erect branching stems bearing bright green, wrinkled, hairless lanceolate leaves wth finely-toothed edges.

The purple flowers, in tight whorls branching from the stem axils, form tapering spikes. *M. spicata crispa* has rounded leaves with curled edges. Spearmint is easily grown from rhizomes cut into pieces 10–15cm long which should be laid horizontally just below the surface of good soil in a moist part of the garden. Mint has grown in parts of the world for thousands of years; although mint sauce now seems almost a British institution, it is not a native plant but was one of the favourite herbs brought here by the Romans. The herbalist Gerard is full of praises for it and one can agree with him that 'its smell rejoiceth the heart of man' and that it does 'stir up the mind to a greedy desire for meat'. The flavour, which complements so well a joint of roast lamb, also helps to digest the meat and its common name of fish mint comes from its doing the same when eaten with oily fish like mackerel or herrings. Put a sprig in the saucepan when cooking greens or pulses, add freshly chopped

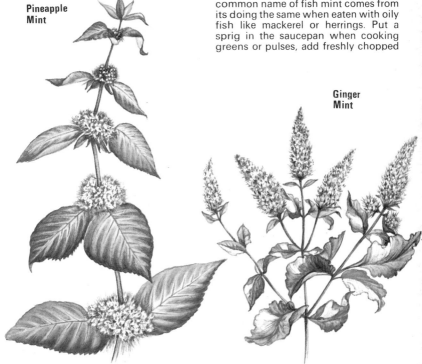

Pineapple
Mint

Ginger
Mint

mint to carrots or courgettes and the tender young tips to salads. Mint can be used in savoury or sweet dishes; as a variation on apple tart, add sultanas, chopped mint and brown sugar to the apples. Use with bananas, apples and nuts with muesli. Freeze mint tips in ice cubes to serve with summer drinks or punch, or float fresh sprigs in the drink. Make mint jelly to serve with meat or fish in the winter months by boiling a handful of fresh, bruised mint in the water, following a basic apple jelly recipe. Cool crushed mint laid across the temples will soothe a headache and is pleasant in hot weather. Bunches hung at open windows may help to discourage flies, and tied under the hot water tap of the bath give a refreshingly fragrant bath, varying the mints for different perfumes.

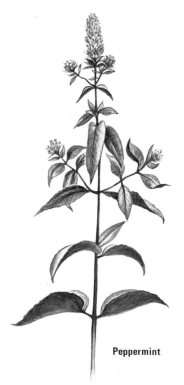

Peppermint

PEPPERMINT
(Black Peppermint)
M. x piperita

One of the most important commercial herbs, yielding peppermint oil for flavouring and medicinal purposes. The plant grows to 60cm with erect, reddish stems and bronze-red pointed, shiny leaves (4–8cm) with serrated edges. Flowers in leaf axils and short tapering spikes. There is no mistaking this mint as true peppermint has a strong smell familiar to everyone. Peppermint tea may be taken for digestive complaints, colds (especially when combined with yarrow and elderflower), hot as a warming beverage, or iced as a clean tasting, refreshing summer drink. If peppermint leaves are crushed and frequently smelled, the 'fumes' from them can help to clear blocked nasal passages. To make delicious after-dinner mints, carefully select some good peppermint leaves, wash and gently dab dry , then brush with lightly beaten white of egg and dust on both sides with icing sugar. Lay the leaves on a cake rack and place in a cool oven to dry and become crisp. Store, when cool, between sheets of greaseproof paper in an airtight container. Pineapple mint leaves, borage, violet and primrose flowers, and red rose petals can quickly be preserved this way. Some peppermint leaves kept in a screw-topped jar of sugar will, like vanilla pods, impart their flavour to the sugar which can then be used in confectionery or baking. White peppermint has green, slightly hairy leaves with coarser serration, but there is little difference in the smell and both are cultivated for the production of oil. The British climate has proved favourable to the commercial production of high quality peppermint oil, although the yield may not equal that from the herb grown on the European continent. A market exists for well dried peppermint to meet the increasing demand for high quality herb teas. The wild *M. aquatica*, with round, purple-tinged leaves, is often found to have a good peppermint smell, being originally a parent plant of the peppermint now cultivated.

PENNYROYAL
(Pudding Grass, Lurk-in-the-ditch)
M. pulegium

A creeping mint rooting from prostrate stems with a dense growth of elliptical shiny bright green leaves (1–1½cm). From mid to late summer the stems turn upwards and bear whorls of pale purple flowers to a height of 10–15cm. There is an upright variety of pennyroyal which has flower stalks 20–30cm. Pieces of rooted stem are easily detached in spring and autumn to start new plants. It gets its name from the latin *pulex*, a flea, because it was used to keep fleas away. Dogs and cats may benefit from having their coats groomed with freshly bruised pennyroyal and some may be put with their bedding. Known in some parts of the country as organy, argony or pudding grass, it was a favourite flavouring for pig's pudding. Pennyroyal flourishes near water and makes a pleasant creeping herb between stones by a pool. If a fragrant herb lawn is desired, it blends unobtrusively into the grass.

CORSICAN MINT
(Spanish Mint)
M. requienii

A prostrate mint forming a close mat with a mass of dull green heart-shaped leaves (to 5mm) and tiny purple flowers, each smaller than a pinhead. The whole plant has a pepperminty smell. On light soils it makes a good carpeting plant in semi-shady areas and on a heavier soil seems to do well in shade or full sun and survives most winters. After severe winters when it seems to have succumbed, it will re-emerge in spring, obviously from self-sown seed. Small clumps will soon spread and can be lifted with soil attached, split and replanted in May or September. It can be walked on with no ill effect and grown between paving, in gravel, rockeries or sink gardens. The tiny flowers, some of the smallest known, give a purple flush to the foliage when in bloom. Though a native of Corsica, *M. requienii* has become naturalized in the United Kingdom and in Ireland.

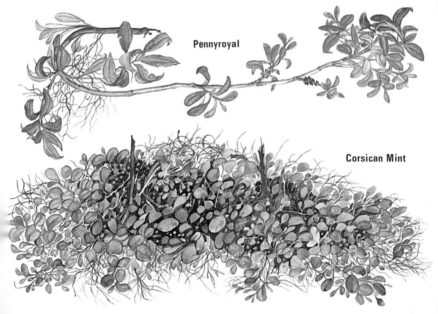

Pennyroyal

Corsican Mint

MOTHERWORT
(Lion's Tail)
Leonurus cardiaca

A hardy perennial, seeding freely. The plant makes a sturdy rootstock from which grow stout square erect stems, sometimes reddish (80–100cm). The basal leaves are palmate and deeply indented; the stem leaves, arranged in opposite pairs, are oblanceolate and divided at the tips, usually into three pointed segments. The flowers, in tight whorls in the axils of the leaves, are pink-lipped and spotted with purple. They are hairy in bud. The calyx is spiny and the flower spike should be handled with care.

Cultivation: from seed sown in spring or autumn or division of root clumps. The plant will grow in most soils. It is an interesting species, with a particularly attractive shape to the early basal leaf growth.

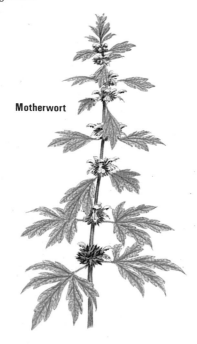

Motherwort

Uses: its name motherwort indicates that the plant's reputation was established from early times as a sedative to calm the nerves of harassed mothers. Modern research shows this herb has alkaloids capable of lowering blood pressure and it may prove to be a valuable plant source for the treatment of cardiac disorders. Its other common name comes from the (somewhat vague) resemblance of the leafy stem to a lion's waving tail.

ROSEMARY
(Dew of the sea)
Rosmarinus officinalis

An evergreen perennial sub-shrub growing to over 1m in sunny sheltered places. The stem becomes woody and the narrow linear dark green leaves are silvery on the undersides. Although the herb flowers most abundantly in spring some flowers may appear from autumn through a mild winter if the shrub is sheltered against a warm wall. The foliage and misty-blue lipped flowers have a strong balsam-like smell which has made rosemary one of the most favoured herbs over many centuries.

Cultivation: rosemary may be grown from seed but the resultant plants may not have the same robustness in surviving winter conditions as plants grown from cuttings taken from healthy stock plants. The bulk of rosemary seed is imported from warmer climates where the herb grows abundantly and the progeny may not have the stamina to flourish in colder conditions. However, if this is appreciated and the young plants are protected from frost pockets and east winds they may well acclimatize and become hardier. Rosemary must have a well-drained soil, which is possible even on clay if sand is added, remembering that the plant's natural habitat is in sandy seaside areas. Cuttings taken in spring will strike quickly and it is wise to nip back the growing tips to make bushy young plants. With mature plants prune as little as possible, just removing broken or unshapely branches.

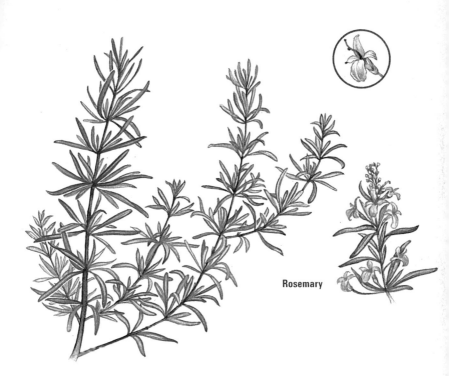

Rosemary

Uses: rosemary oil and waters have been used extensively in cosmetic and medicinal preparations for thousands of years. It has digestive, tonic and antiseptic properties and has been used as a gargle and taken as a tea for nausea, headaches and as a sedative. Externally the oil is used as an embrocation by sufferers from aching joints and neuralgia. Rosemary is also an excellent tonic for the hair. A handful of stems should be put in a jug and boiling water poured over them. The jug is covered and left to cool and the strained liquid massaged into the scalp and used as a final rinse after washing the hair. As rosemary is evergreen it is usually possible to pick it fresh from the bush, even in winter, so drying is unnecessary. It can be rubbed into and cooked

with lamb, pork, chicken and fish. Some sprigs kept in a jar of sugar will impart its flavour for use in apple pies, cakes and biscuits. In winter mulled cider with rosemary and cloves makes a heart-warming beverage for those coming in from the cold. An orange with short tips of rosemary pushed into the skin (a fine skewer will make the holes) and tied with ribbon makes an aromatic pomander-like 'visiting gift'. In warmer parts of the country the prostrate rosemary *(R. prostratus)* will drape elegantly over walls and down steps. For less balmy areas it is best grown in a pot and brought indoors for winter shelter. Similar treatment should be given to the gilded rosemary *(R. aurea variegata)*, whose leaves are splashed with gold colour.

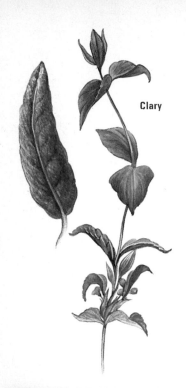

Clary

CLARY
(Bluebeard)
Salvia horminum
An annual forming a group of basal hairy ovate leaves (7cm), with rough pitted surfaces and finely crenate edges. The square hairy stems (to 50cm) terminate in several opposite pairs of deep blue bracts. The lipped flowers come from the axils of the leaves in pairs.

Cultivation: by seed in spring. It will grow in an open position in most soils and will flower on into the autumn with the bracts making a colourful display.

Uses: mainly a decorative garden plant, interesting in flower arrangements and liked by bees. Winemakers may care to know that it is said to improve the inebriating quality of wine. In the past it was one of the herbs used for snuff.

SAGE
Salvia officinalis
A familiar perennial herb in most gardens, growing as a bush (to 90cm across) with woody rootstocks and

The foliage of these sages complement each other and can also be used for culinary purposes.

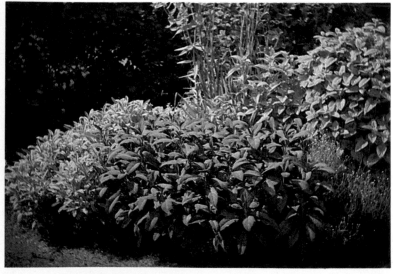

much-branched stems bearing oblong grey-green entire leaves with wrinkled surfaces.

Cultivation: there are two types of common sage, narrow-leaved and broad-leaved. Narrow-leaved sage is grown from seed and has more pointed, rather greyer leaves than the broad-leaved type which does not produce viable seed and must be propagated vegetatively. The flowering narrow-leaved sage is decorative, with spikes of purple flowers. Broad-leaved sage produces good crops of leaf for drying; its less intense flavour is preferred for culinary purposes in many cases.

Uses: the name salvia, coming from the Latin for 'to save', indicates the virtues attributed to this herb of restoring health and saving from sickness. It was extolled in a proverb: 'He that would live for aye must eat sage in May'. In addition to its culinary use in stuffings, sauces and salads, it can be taken as a wholesome tea throughout the year.

RED SAGE
S. officinalis purpurascens

Many centuries ago someone observed on a common green sage bush shoots out of character with the usual growth. These were detached and propagated vegetatively, and have come down to us as red sage (though the foliage is in fact purple and green). *Salvia tricolor*, with a white edging around the leaves, is choice but not quite so hardy.

Cultivation: by cuttings or layering.

Uses: an infusion of red sage is an antiseptic gargle for sore throats.

GOLDEN VARIEGATED SAGE
S. officinalis icterina

Another variety of sage with gold and green variegated leaves. Should be planted in full sunlight. In small gardens these decorative sages might well replace the common green sage as they can be used for culinary and simple medicinal purposes in the same way.

CLARY SAGE
(Clear Eye)
Salvia sclarea

Botanically this handsome plant is a biennial, but if the flower stalks are removed in autumn it will sometimes

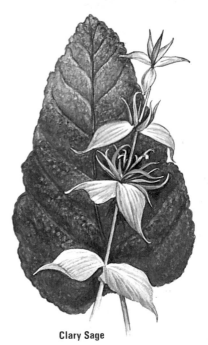

Clary Sage

persist for 3 or 4 years. In the first year it forms a rosette of broad cordate leaves, and in the second year the flowering stems grow to 100–150cm, the leaves becoming smaller towards the top. The branching flower spikes are drooping in bud and become erect as the flowers open. The small-lipped flowers, pink-white or purple-white, are insignificant compared with the large pink bracts which give the plant its striking effect.

Cultivation: by seed sown in spring or autumn. This plant looks best against a dark background. Because of its strong smell it should not be used in flower arrangements.

Uses: clary sage oil is used as a fixative for perfumes. Its common name 'clear eye' may come from the word clary, or more likely from its use to remove obstructions from the eyes. The mucilage from the soaked seeds helps to do this, and to soothe the inflamed eyes. The young leaves dipped in batter were cooked as fritters.

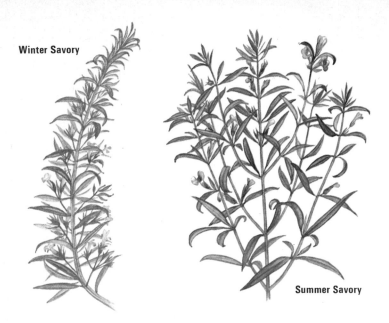

Winter Savory

Summer Savory

WINTER SAVORY
(Bean herb)
Satureja montana
A small, hardy , evergreen, bushy herb of compact habit (to 30cm). The branching stems bear opposite pairs of linear, dark green leaves (1–2cm) and from midsummer small white or pale mauve flowers.
Cultivation: from seed, cuttings, layering or division. Mountainous regions are savory's natural habitat, so a well-drained poorish soil will suit it and in such a position it will persist for many years if trimmed back into shape after flowering and given a compost mulch in autumn. It should be given plenty of space, not overcrowded by other plants.
Uses: as a savoury herb in soups, casseroles and in salads. Blended with a little grated horseradish, it goes well with fish, particularly trout. As we put sprigs of mint with peas, in Europe savory is added when cooking beans for, as its alternative name indicates, it complements all types of beans. This perennial savory is an excellent alternative to the annual summer savory.

SUMMER SAVORY
Satureja hortensis
An annual herb with erect, soft, sparsely branching stems (30cm) and long internodes. The leaves ($1\frac{1}{2}$–2cm) are light green and there are pale pink flowers in the axils of the leaves.
Cultivation: from seed sown indoors in April or outside in May. The plant will not survive frost in spring or autumn. It is one of the annual herbs which respond to being potted and brought indoors in early autumn to keep growth going. If winter savory is being grown from seed it is a good idea to sow summer savory also, so that the annual herb can be used while the perennial plants are getting established. Although the alliterative summer savory is usually the one mentioned in recipes it seems to have little to commend it compared with the perennial winter savory.
Uses: the same as for winter savory. Savory vinegar made with wine vinegar is good served with fish or used in salad dressings. It provides a good digestive tea and helps to soothe the irritation from insect bites.

SELF HEAL
(Prunella)
Prunella vulgaris
A widely distributed plant common in many parts of the world, spreading rapidly by virtue of its probing rhizomes and abundant seed. The square stems (to 50cm) bear ovate, entire or slightly-toothed leaves (3–6cm), narrowing as they progress up the stem. The mauve-pink flowers are in curious, tightly-packed whorls, the florets opening irregularly from midsummer.

Cultivation: by detached rooted rhizomes, division of the plant or seed, in spring.

Uses: used as a strong infusion, this herb has a well-founded reputation as an effective styptic. It has also been used as a diuretic, a gargle for mouth infections and as an external wash for skin complaints. In a wild part of the garden it makes useful ground cover.

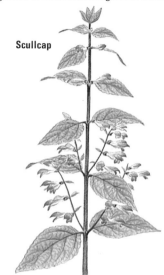

Scullcap

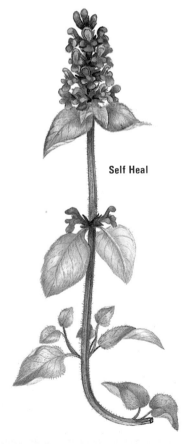

Self Heal

SCULLCAP
(Virginian scullcap, Mad dog scullcap)
Scutellaria lateriflora
There are innumerable scullcaps growing from 8cm to over 1m. In Britain there are two native species, common scullcap *(S. galericulata)* and lesser scullcap *(S. minor)*, and hybrids may occur. *S. lateriflora* is often cultivated and has a bushy habit: before it flowers it looks much like lemon balm. Fibrous roots form a sturdy rootstock and the erect stems (to 60cm) bear opposite, ovate or elliptical, downy, toothed leaves of mid-green. The flower stalks branch from the axils of the leaves and are arranged as one-sided racemes of violet blue. The seeds are in an interesting lidded capsule which later dries, splits and disperses them when they are ripe.

Cultivation: by seed or division of the rootstock in spring. The plant does well in most soils in a sunny position.

Uses: An infusion is used to calm the nerves and as a tonic. At one time it was held in such high repute that it was given as a treatment for hydrophobia, hence the name Mad dog scullcap.

THYME
(Common Thyme)
Thymus vulgaris
A small bushy perennial (to 30cm) with much-branched stems becoming woody. There are two types, one with lanceolate grey-green leaves, the other with ovate green leaves (5–8cm). In late spring the bushes are covered with masses of flower spikes bearing whorls of purple florets.

Cultivation: by seed which usually produces the grey-green narrow-leaved type or by cuttings, layering and division of root from bushes showing the broader green leaves. Thyme needs a well-drained soil and open position and should be sheared of the dead flowering growth if it has not been cut for culinary or medicinal use. The herb may be cut for drying in May before the flowers open and again in autumn, after which compost should be spread around the plants.

Uses: a well-known herb for flavouring stuffings, sausages, soups and salads. It has valuable antiseptic properties as a medicinal herb. An infusion should be drunk for colds, coughs, throat infections and used to bathe skin eruptions.

LEMON THYME
Thymus citriodorus
Similar in habit and growth to common thyme but it does not always come true from seed and is better propagated from cuttings, layering or division. This plant has a true lemon scent and can replace a lemon to flavour stuffings, makes a refreshing lemon drink and can be dried for pot pourri.

SILVER THYME
Thymus vulgaris 'Silver Posy'
A small bush thyme with attractive silver-edged leaves, the undersides of which are tinged with pink. It grows like common thyme and has the same scent. It should be grown in full sun and trimmed into shape after flowering to prevent the growth becoming straggly. Mulch with compost in the autumn.

SILVER THYME
T. citriodorus 'Silver Queen'
A cultivar with lemon-scented foliage but too prone to revert to its green-leaved parent, lemon thyme. Growing on very poor soil may delay this

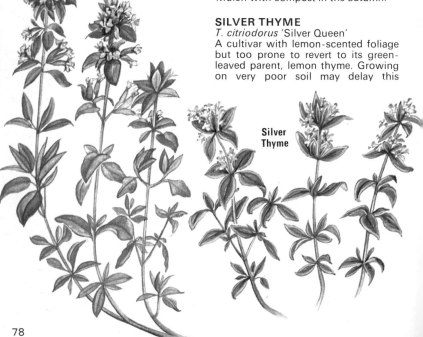

Wild Thyme

Silver Thyme

78

reversion, but if constant silver foliage is required it is better to grow the reliable 'Silver Posy' which seldom reverts.

GOLDEN THYME
Thymus aureus
A semi-prostrate cushion thyme with golden foliage all the year round and a sharp scent similar to that of common thyme. Because of its colour it is sometimes mistakenly called lemon thyme. Easily propagated by cuttings or division of root and will self sow, usually coming true.

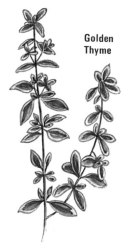

Golden Thyme

GOLDEN LEMON THYME
T. citriodorus aureus
A bush thyme similar to those with silver variegated foliage and with lemon-scented foliage, but having an unfortunate tendency to revert back to the green lemon thyme. Grow in poor soil and remove any growth showing reversion.

CREEPING THYMES
Thymus serpyllum sps.
A delightful group of creeping or carpeting herbs with a variety of leaf shapes and textures and flower colours. They can be used with effect on rockeries, to hang over walls and down steps, in sink and trough gardens, between paving stones and in gravel walks, or massed as an alternative 'lawn'. Soil should be light, drainage good and the situation exposed to maximum sunlight.

Cultivation: there are many named cultivars and innumerable hybrids. If grown from seed it is impossible to guarantee that the plants will come true, but cuttings, layering or division will ensure this. It is usually possible to obtain the following variety of plants: *T. serp. coccineus* with deep red flowers; *T. serp. albus* light green foliage and white flowers; *T. serp. doerflerii, lanuginosus* or 'Pink Chintz', all of which have grey woolly foliage and pink or purple flowers; *T. serp. Bressingham seedling*, a robust quickly spreading thyme for carpeting; and *T. serp. Herba Barona*, a caraway-scented thyme which used to be rubbed on barons of beef to improve the flavour, or possibly to mask the fact that the meat was not as fresh as it might be!

Uses: because of their prostrate habit and small foliage, creeping thymes are not as serviceable for culinary use as the bush thymes but visually they can give much pleasure.

Creeping thymes spread rapidly pouring their colour between paving and over stones

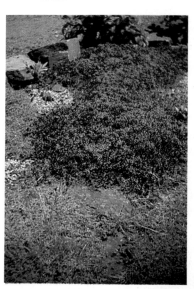

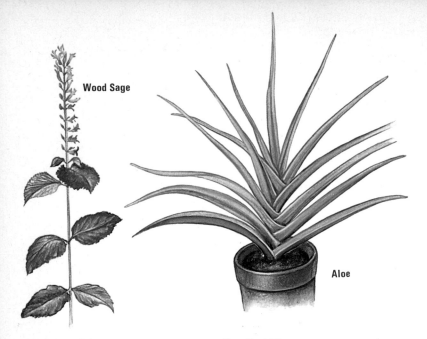

Wood Sage

Aloe

WOOD SAGE
Teucrium scorodonia
A perennial herb with creeping root-stock and stems to 45cm. The dull green, ovate, sage-like leaves (2–4cm) have wrinkled surfaces and crenate edges. The small flowers are a pale yellowish-green – and are arranged in pairs on one side of the leafless stalks, in branching spikes. The specific name *scorodonia* implies that the plant has a garlic smell, although a smell of hops would be more accurate.

Cultivation: from seed or division of root in sprng. It will grow in most soils, but does well in semi-shade.

Uses: wood sage warrants a place in a herb bed because its basal foliage usually survives the winter and its unusual flowers – of a colour un-characteristic in labiates – give it interest, particularly to flower arran-gers. It was used in the making of ales before hops were introduced and is considered a good bitter tonic and blood cleanser. An infusion made from the leaves and flowering tops may be of benefit to sufferers from rheumatic complaints. It is used externally to bathe or poultice skin troubles.

Family Liliaceae

ALOE
Aloe vera (A. Barbadensis)
A succulent tropical plant forming clusters of fleshy pale green leaves, which as they mature become prickly at the edges. After 3–4 years it may produce leafless stems bearing racemes of orange-red tubular flowers.

Cultivation: this plant must be grown as a greenhouse or house plant in a light gritty compost to ensure good drainage; it rots if it becomes too wet. Small plantlets will develop at the base of the plant and these can be detached to grow on in other pots.

Uses: aloe is an ancient plant with a long history of medicinal use and it is still being researched for its use in the treatment of severe burns, serious skin problems and a wide range of other complaints. Grown as a pot plant on the kitchen window sill it may prove helpful in coping with minor domestic mishaps such as burns, cuts and scratches. A piece of leaf sliced through and the cut side instantly applied to an injury is emollient and will cool, seal and help to heal.

CHIVES
Allium schoenoprasum

An easily-grown perennial herb with fibrous roots and grass-like tubular tapering leaves (15–25cm). The leafless flower stems terminate in bunched heads of thrift-like purple florets.

Cultivation: from seed sown in spring or autumn or by dividing the clumps into 6–10 bulbs for replanting. It will grow well in most soils and although the plants die down in late autumn they usually reappear with the first mild weather of February. When the seeds are black and ripe in late summer they may be shaken out of the flowerheads and sown in shallow drills. In late autumn pull up some fine soil either side to protect them for the winter.

Uses: the tender green leaves of chives give a mild onion flavour. They can be chopped into almost any kind of salad, or used with egg, cheese, fish and vegetable dishes to flavour or garnish. The newly opened flowerheads are also edible. They may be split into individual florets and added to salads and added to rice or soups just before serving. Giant chives grows about twice as big as the common chives and the bulbs can be pulled like spring onions. Chives leaves do not keep their flavour and colour as well as other herbs when dried but they freeze well.

GARLIC
Allium sativum

A perennial compound bulb, although usually grown as an annual like onions and shallots. The bulb is made up of many bulblets known as 'cloves' held together within a paper sheath. The leaves are flat and linear, tapering to about 30cm. The flower stalk in late summer has a terminal head of white florets and tiny bulbils.

Cultivation: cloves separated from the parent bulb should be planted about 10cm apart in good, well-drained soil in a sunny position. On light soils planting should be done in autumn, on heavy soils in early spring as soon as the soil can be worked. The bulbs will be ready for harvesting in early autumn. If some are left in the ground to grow on they will provide useful garlic-flavoured green foliage.

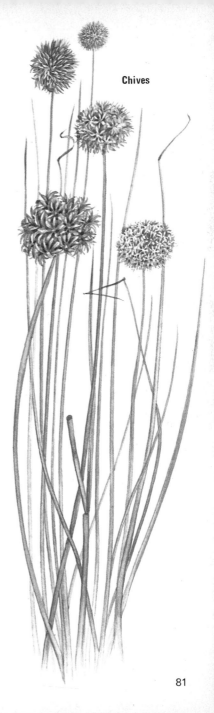

Chives

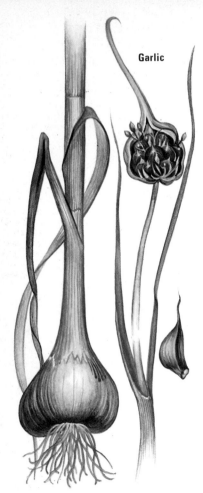

Garlic

robbed the dead and dying of their valuables. In cooking, garlic enhances many dishes and loses its strong smell. If it gives offence when eaten raw, parsley, mint, sweet cicely or peppermint will help to freshen the breath. It is rich in vitamins and undoubtedly a health-promoting herb.

GARLIC CHIVES
Allium tuberosum
A perennial much like chives, growing in clumps but with flat linear leaves (30–45cm) and terminal umbels of white star-shaped florets. Garlic chives may be grown from seed or division of the clumps in spring or autumn and can be used in the same ways as chives.

RAMSONS
Allium ursinum
A perennial with broad shiny leaves similar to lily of the valley, but easily distinguished by the strong garlic smell when the leaves are bruised. When the plant is in flower, with its attractive umbels of white star-like stalked florets carried on a stem to 30cm, the

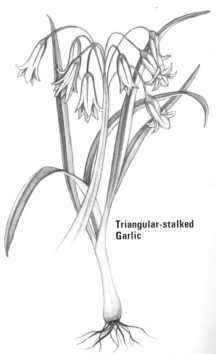

Triangular-stalked Garlic

Uses: for thousands of years, the valuable antiseptic properties of garlic have protected people from a number of unpleasant infections. It destroys certain harmful bacteria and is beneficial in combating coughs, colds, bronchial conditions and skin complaints. A cut clove of garlic is an effective first aid remedy pressed on to cuts and scratches. It was an important ingredient of a recipe known as 'the vinegar of the four thieves' which gave immunity to a band of infamous rascals who, at a time of plague in Marseilles, unmistakable garlic smell pervades the area. In light woodland it is pretty enough to be allowed to naturalize. *Allium moly* has umbels of buttercup-yellow florets and dull grey-green broad leaves. It is a welcome late spring flowering bulb in many gardens. The round bulbs, about the size of a hazel nut, should be planted in groups in autumn where it will be welcome if it multiplies and spreads. The yellow florets are decorative in salads and give a delicate garlic flavour.

TRIANGULAR-STALKED GARLIC
Allium triquetrum
An interesting perennial garlic (to 30cm) with three-sided leaves and dainty flowerheads of drooping white bells. Each petal is marked with a green line, and the florets are suspended on long stalks from one side of the triangular stem. The bulbs multiply rapidly and the leaves can be used for flavouring.

TREE ONION
(Egyptian onion)
Allium cepa var. *proliferum*
Alliums are rich in the variety they offer and tree onion may be considered an exhibitionist in the group. At the top of sturdy hollow stems (to 50cm) heads of small onions develop, usually 4–6 in number. Sometimes another slender stem grows through them, again surmounted with tiny onions. If the first tier is thinned to 4 and secondary growth discouraged, the onions can be used for soups or when only small quantities are needed in cooking. As the plant ripens the stems turn straw-coloured and bend over, setting the young onions at soil level to restart the cycle of growth. These young onions, put several in a pot on a kitchen window sill, will sprout freely and provide winter onion green over a long period. They are more successful than chives, which if treated in this way tend to get thin and wispy.

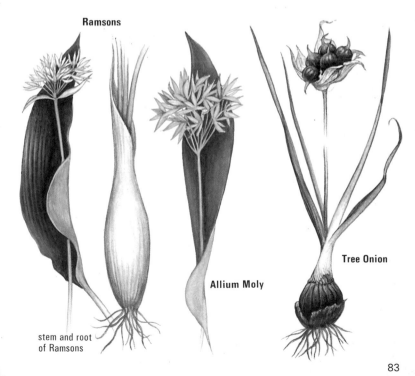

Ramsons

Allium Moly

Tree Onion

stem and root of Ramsons

Family Linaceae

LINSEED FLAX
Linum usitatissimum

This annual grows on slender stems to about 120cm with blue-green, lanceolate, alternate, stalkless leaves (3–5cm). The obovate, 5-petalled flowers are sky-blue and grow in loose terminal corymbs.

Cultivation: by seed sown in late spring on good well-drained soil. Flax is best sown where it is to flower as it does not transplant well.

Uses: this delicate-looking plant has been an invaluable element in the economy of many civilizations since at least 5000 BC. Cloth spun from flax has been found in ancient tombs. It was used for clothing and hangings in houses and temples; for sails and the thread for fishnets; for ropes and bow strings; and, knotted with tow, stuffed into the cracks of boats. To make cloth, the flax was soaked, dried in the sun, tried into bundles, and then, as a medieval account has it, 'knockyd, beten, rodded and gnodded, ribbed and heklyd and at last sponne'. Equally important is its yield of oil. Commercial crops of linseed have been grown in many parts of the world for use in paints, varnish and putty, as a fattening food for cattle and in veterinary medicine. Externally it may be used as a poultice for boils, inflammation and wounds. There is an annual red-flowered flax *(L. rubrum)* which has rich crimson flowers and blooms over a long period. Sow seed in late spring.

PERENNIAL FLAX
Linum perenne

An erect bushy perennial (to about 60cm) with linear leaves and rather paler blue flowers than the annual flax.

Cultivation: by seed in well-drained soil. Should not be moved, so sow the seed where you want the plant to grow. The flowers open new each morning and fade by evening, keeping up a succession of blooms for many weeks.

Uses: an ornamental plant providing patches of soft blue. The seeds contain oil but it is not as highly esteemed commercially as that of the common flax.

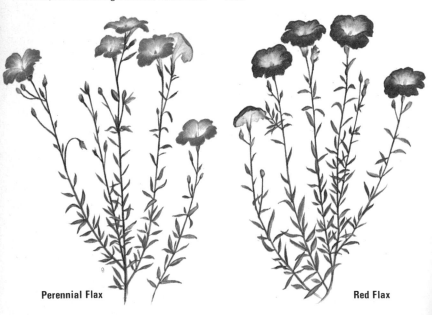

Perennial Flax   **Red Flax**

Family Lauraceae

BAY
(Sweet Bay, Noble laurel)
Laurus nobilis
A shrub or small tree with dull green or dark red woody stems. The shiny dark green alternate leaves are ovate or broad lanceolate with wavy edges (to 14cm). The plant flowers irregularly with small clusters of unisexual yellowish blossoms appearing in the axils of the leaves in early summer.

Cultivation: bay can be grown from seed but it is a long process. It is best grown from cuttings, taken in late summer and potted up in a sharp sand or gritty compost and overwintered in a cold greenhouse (in frost free areas the pots may be sunk into soil under a west wall). Low-growing stems may be layered and pegged down from the parent bush. Young bay trees should be given protection from east winds and in areas where severe winters are expected it is best to grow small trees in tubs or large pots so that they can be brought under cover for winter. With established trees severe weather may damage the top growth but the tree will usually shoot again from the base.

Uses: bay trees are used as ornamental feature plants either as natural bushes or trained into various shapes. The aroma of a crushed bay leaf is very pleasant and is used in cooking with fish, lamb, marinades and soups, for bouquet garni and milk puddings. Bay leaves do not retain good colour after drying and if possible fresh leaves should always be used. The noble laurel was a symbol of achievement in ancient times and branches of bay were woven into crowns for victors at the games and to celebrate great artistic successes (hence the term 'poet laureate'). It was thought to have protective and antiseptic virtues and the bruised leaves were smelled or the branches burned where there was infection. Care must be taken not to confuse the leaves of *L. nobilis* with those of the Cherry laurel *(Prunus laurocerasus)* with leaves serrated at the edges, and Mountain laurel *(Kalmia latifolia)* with flowers that look as if they might have been made of piped fondant icing. Both of these plants can be poisonous.

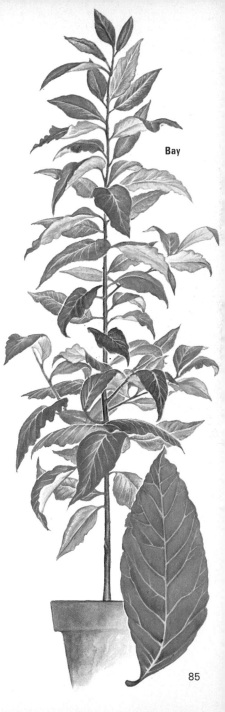

Bay

85

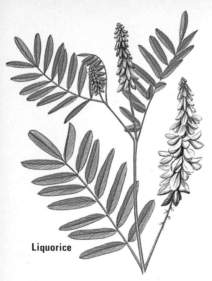

Liquorice

Family Leguminoseae

LIQUORICE
Glycyrrhiza glabra
An erect hairless perennial plant (60–120cm) which first establishes vertical slender taproots and then develops horizontal rhizomes which spread extensively. The branching stems bear oblong pinnate leaflets and terminal racemes of pale purple small pea flowers.

Cultivation: this herb needs a humus-rich soil but good drainage. It requires moisture but should not get water-logged. Rhizomes can be removed from the parent plant in autumn, cut into 8cm pieces and replanted in good soil. The new growth does not emerge until late in spring and the ground around the plants should not be disturbed until growth shows, but a dressing of compost in spring and manure in autumn will encourage strong growth. When the herb is grown commercially, the roots are not harvested until the plant is four years old.

Uses: liquorice has been a herb of great commercial importance over thousands of years, widely used for flavouring and medicinal purposes. It has been used in the processing of tobacco, in ales and stouts and to mask the flavour of unpleasant medicines. It is a good digestive and combined with linseed, honey and lemon makes a soothing drink for troublesome coughs. At one time it was grown on a large scale in England, chiefly in the Pontefract area of Yorkshire and sold in quantity as a confection known as Pontefract or Pomfrey cakes, flat discs of liquorice about 2cm across.

MELILOT
(Yellow Sweet Clover)
Melilotus officinalis
A biennial bushy plant with branching stems and trifoliate oblong serrated leaflets. The flower stems come from the axils of the leaves and form racemes of small yellow pea flowers, favoured by bees.

Cultivation: from seed sown in spring or autumn. Will self-sow freely after flowering and does well in most soils.

Uses: to flavour alcoholic beverages, cheese and as an ingredient of herbal tobacco. The dried herb smells deliciously of new-mown hay and is pleasant to have in bowls in a room or to add to pot pourri. It was also used as a strewing herb because of its wholesome scent. Modern research has pointed to its making a contribution in the prevention of thrombosis.

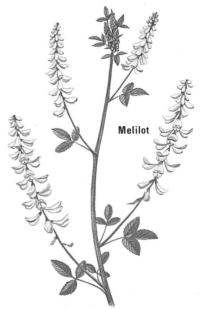

Melilot

Family Malvaceae

COMMON MALLOW
Malva sylvestris

A rather straggling perennial herb, either prostrate and spreading or erect and bushy, according to habitat. The basal leaves are palmate and crinkly, sometimes spotted at base, and becoming more deeply lobed on the stems. The flowers have 5 notched petals, rosy-pink with purple stripes, twisted in bud stage and in a hairy calyx. The seeds, or nutlets, are arranged in a flat circular disc. Aptly named 'cheeses' by country children, they are edible and have a pleasant hazelnut flavour.

Cultivation: this plant grows readily from seed or by pieces of the rootstock pulled off at the base of the plant and replanted. In the wild it is a low-growing plant found on roadsides and dry banks, but cultivated plants will reach 80–90cm in height, making a handsome, bushy plant massed with flowers over a long period.

Uses: all mallows have emollient properties and are useful to draw and soothe boils, inflamed areas or unhealthy sores. The tender young stalks can be cut into pea-sized pieces and cooked as a vegetable in spring with mint, chives, savory, lovage or some other flavouring herb as they are rather bland on their own.

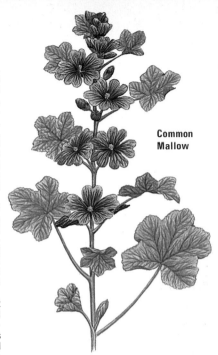

Common
Mallow

With its rose-pink coloured flowers, musk mallow grows wild on sunny roadside banks.

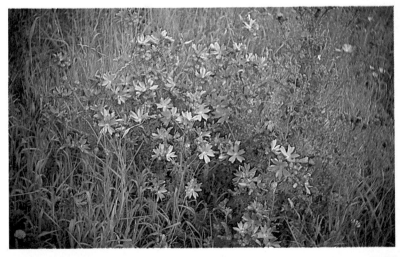

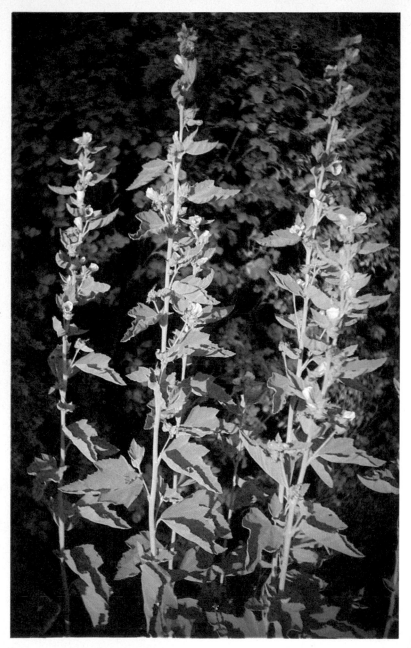

MARSHMALLOW
Althaea officinalis

A hardy perennial herb with long whitish taproots and erect pithy stems (to 100cm). The soft downy grey-green leaves are broad ovate, pointed and slightly lobed. The 5-petalled pale mauve-pink flowers (2–4cm) develop in small clusters from the axils of the leaves.

Cultivation: from seed or division of root showing a growing point. Its name indicates this plant's preference for damp places, its natural habitat being marshy areas, but it will grow successfully in moisture-retaining soil in gardens – a charming combination of soft velvety foliage and delicate flowers.

Uses: the whole plant and particularly the root contains abundant mucilage and in the past this was used for confectionary, but the sweets sold as marshmallows today have no connection with this herb. Medicinally it may be used with equal safety internally or externally as an emollient for inflammation, ulcers, burns, for cleansing wounds and to soothe chest complaints. A soothing drink for children's coughs can be made by chopping and soaking 50gr (1¾oz) of scraped marshmallow root in water for 30 minutes, bringing slowly to the boil and simmering very gently for 5 minutes. Cool, strain and add a good teaspoonful of honey and the juices of an orange and half a lemon. Sip as needed. The leaves can be used as a poultice for bruises and sprains, and an ointment made from the root and/or leaves will reduce inflammation. Because of its reputation for cleansing unhealthy wounds it became known as Mortification root.

Family Onagraceae

EVENING PRIMROSE
Oenothera biennis

An edible biennial which in the first year forms a rosette of elliptic, slightly-toothed leaves and a stumpy taproot. In the second year this sends up a flowering stem (80–100cm) which

The pale pink flowers and soft, velvety grey-green leaves of marshmallow look well against a dark background.

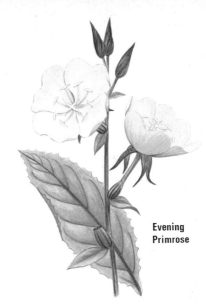

Evening Primrose

branches and shows reddish colour on the stem and midribs of the lanceolate leaves. Racemes of flowers come from the axils of the leaves. The flower bud is encased in a hairy red calyx which splits to reveal the broad yellow petals, delicately scented in the evenings.

Cultivation: from seed sown in spring or autumn. It will grow in quite poor conditions and most soils; and self-sows freely.

Uses: the first year leaves can be used in salads while tender and the roots grated and eaten raw or cooked as vegetables. By the time the plant comes into flower the roots are coarse and stringy. Evening primrose is an American native plant but has naturalized here since it was introduced in the 17th century, and may be found growing wild on roadsides and in seaside areas. From a medicinal point of view it may excite more interest than it has done in the light of modern research into its constituents and their potential for preventing heart ailments. Ornamental varieties with larger flowers are *O. Lamarkiana* and a dwarf cultivar *O. missouriensis*, suitable for rockeries, which gives a lasting display of yellow flowers on short, spreading stems.

Family Papilionaceae

GOAT'S RUE
Galega officinalis

A strong-growing hardy perennial of bushy habit (to 1m) with hollow branching stems bearing lanceolate pinnate leaflets (to 4cm). The long flower stalks terminate in racemes of small white pea-like flowers in summer. There are cultivars with blue and lilac-pink flowers.

Cultivation: by seed or division of the rootstocks in spring or autumn. Goat's rue does well on a heavy soil as it flourishes where there is plenty of moisture. When in flower it is a splendid sight and needs an area of about 70cm for its spread.

Uses: the generic name *galega*, meaning milk, indicates its reputation for stimulating the secretion of milk when taken as an infusion of the fresh plant. The juice of the herb is used to clot milk for junket or cheesemaking. In the past it was employed in a footbath 'to refresh the feet of those tired with overmuch walking'.

Family Polygonaceae

SORREL
(Sour sauce)
Rumex acetosa

A hardy perennial herb with taproot and reddish stems (80–100cm) terminating in whorled spikes of tiny red-green flowers, ripening to rich brown seeds.

Cultivation: seeds of the broadleaved cultivated sorrel germinate quickly sown out of doors in late spring and plants should not be allowed to flower if maximum leaf is required. It will grow well in most soils and conditions. This broad-leaved type is sometimes called French sorrel, but so also, confusingly, is the small Buckler's sorrel *(Rumex scutatus)* with broad reniform, lobed leaves, which grows only to about

Goat's Rue

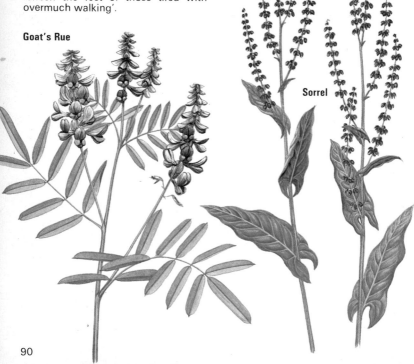

Sorrel

50cm. Wild sorrel *(R. acetosella)* is found in open meadows and grassland and recognized by its deeply cut spear-shaped leaves. All sorrels have the sharp apple flavour which is refreshingly thirst-quenching when chewed on a hot summer day and delicious added to salads or used as a sauce, as an alternative to apple sauce, with pork, duck or goose. The sharp flavour is due to the oxalic acids the plants contain and too much should not be eaten by anyone with a tendency to gout or rheumatic complaints. To make sorrel sauce, take a couple of handfuls of leaves, wash and finely chop them, then gently simmer them in the water still adhering to them. To $\frac{1}{4}$ pint (150ml) of the juice that forms add $\frac{3}{4}$ pint

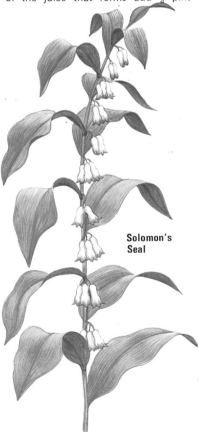

Solomon's Seal

(450ml) of stock and a couple of sprigs of chopped sweet cicely. Blend a dessertspoonful of flour with enough cold milk to make it creamy and add this to the herbs and stock, with a knob of butter and a scrape of nutmeg. Bring gently to the boil and stir for 2 or 3 minutes then remove from the heat and if possible put through a blender or liquidiser.

SOLOMON'S SEAL
Polygonatum multiflorum
A hairless perennial growing from thick rhizomes. The stems are erect at first and then arching, carrying the ribbed, broad lanceolate, alternate leaves growing from the upper sides of the stems. From the base of the leaves, underneath the stems, hang groups of 2–7 stalked, waisted, bell-shaped white flowers with green markings. The berries that follow are black.

Cultivation: fresh seed sown in autumn and left in the cold ground over the winter will stratify and germinate in spring. In autumn, after the plant has died back, or in very early spring, the rhizomes can be lifted and cut so that each piece for replanting retains a growing point or bud. This is an attractive plant to naturalize in a semi-shady shrubby or woody area; humus and leaf-mould in the soil will encourage it to spread.

Uses: plants that are happy in shade are welcome in most gardens, particularly when they have the elegance of solomon's seal. It may prove effective, pounded fresh or dried and ground, as a poultice to cure inflammation and bruises. An infusion was used as a cosmetic wash to remove blemishes on the skin. Herbs, often containing antiseptic oils, infused and used as facial washes or to bathe the body can seldom do anything but good. Their popularity and the virtues ascribed to them in days when cleanliness was neither as easily achieved nor thought as important as in recent times, causes one to conjecture that it may not have been the potency of any particular herb that seemed so beneficial, but that any wholesome herb, infused and used for washing, made the toilette a more pleasurable exercise and was bound to improve the condition of the skin.

Family Plantaginaceae

GREATER PLANTAIN
(Rat-tail plantain)
Plantago major

A scentless perennial forming a basal rosette of broad ovate, prominently-veined leaves (to 15cm). The stems (15–20cm) have long spikes of tiny yellowish flowers with purple anthers (conspicuous for wind pollination).

Cultivation and uses: This 'weed' herb should only be allowed in a wild area of the garden as it is seriously invasive. It has spread to many parts of the world and is widely used in simple medicinal treatments. The cooling, slightly astringent property of the leaves makes it effective applied directly, as pulped foliage, to burns and sores, and it may help to arrest bleeding of minor wounds. Rubbed on insect bites, stings and nettle stings it gives relief from irritation. An ointment made from a combination of plantain and chickweed is soothing for skin eruptions. The seeds yield mucilage and an infusion made from them, sweetened with honey, is a safe drink for children troubled with coughs. Chaucer, Shakespeare and Longfellow all mention its healing powers and the American Indians used it as an antidote to snake bites. The young leaves can be eaten but are salty and a little bitter to taste, and so more palatable in mixed salads. They can be cooked as a green vegetable. The other familiar 'weed' in the large plantain family is ribwort *(P. lanceolata)* with narrow, deeply-ribbed leaves and short spikes of green and brown flowerheads.

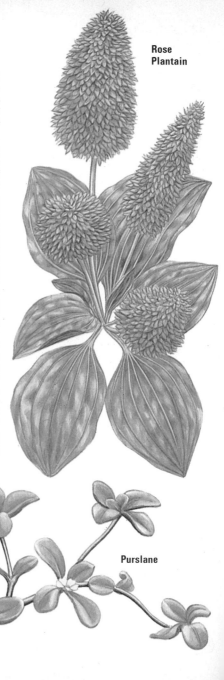

Rose Plantain

Purslane

ROSE PLANTAIN
P. major rosulatus

A less common all-green plantain interesting to flower and foliage arrangers. The basal leaves are similar to those of broad-leaved *(P. major)* but tend to curl inwards a little at the edges. The stems (to 30cm) bear a variety of flowerhead shapes, some like a green cabbage rose, others conical, circular or mushroom-shaped and they seem to develop in a haphazard manner with different shapes on the same plant. The florets are hidden, sheltered in the leaf-like bracts, but the plant seeds freely and should be grown where it is possible to keep seedlings under control. A fungicide spray early in the season is advised as the plant sometimes falls victim to mildew which gives it a shabby look and if not treated it is best dug up and burned.

Family Portulaceae

PURSLANE
Portulaca oleracea

A fleshy semi-prostrate annual with pinkish stems (to 15cm) and succulent obovate leaves (to 2cm). The incon-spicuous yellowish flowers bloom in late summer.

Cultivation and uses: an easily grown annual in a dry, sunny position. Makes a useful edging to a salad bed and is one of those agreeable cut-and-come-again herbs. It is rich in vitamin C and a good skin tonic and diuretic.

Family Primulaceae

COWSLIP
Primula veris

A favourite country wild flower which must be protected and tended to ensure that it continues growing and seeding in the areas natural to it. A perennial with oblong, ovate, veined leaves with crinkly surfaces, forming first a rosette and then bearing the nodding umbel-like clusters of orange-yellow flowers in a tubular light green calyx.

Cultivation and uses: by seed in autumn or division of root clumps in spring or autumn. Seeds of many wild plants can now be obtained from reputable seed firms. Young leaves and petals can be used in salads, but it is good to let cowslips naturalize somewhere in the garden just for the pleasure of their presence.

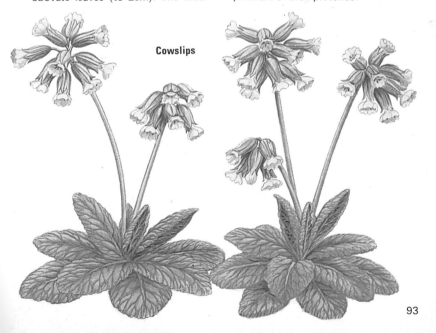

Cowslips

PRIMROSE

Primula vulgaris

Well-known perennial spring flower with obovate leaves, deeply veined and wrinkled, and hairy on the underside. The single pale yellow flowers, which grow on a reddish hairy stalk, are tubular at the base and divide into 5 heart-shaped petals.

Cultivation: by seed or division of the rootstock. Wild plants should not be dug up (seed can be obtained from almost any seed firm). Hybrids of cowslips, oxlips, primroses and polyanthus will readily occur, and particularly interesting ones can be propagated by division of rootstock to ensure that the progeny comes true. Planted near silver foliage *Primula* 'Garryarde Guinevere' is a lovely surprise in spring with its red-bronze leaves and blush-pink primrose flowers. Owing to the enthusiasm of a few specialists it is once again possible to find double-flowered primroses, a delight of the old cottage gardens, which were in danger of becoming lost.

Uses: the tender young leaves and flowers can be used in salads, as they were in the magnificent 'sallets' of Elizabethan times which included 20 or 30 different kinds of leaves, flowers, roots and herbs. The flowers may be candied, using the method described for peppermint leaves, and primrose

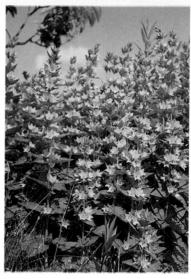

Yellow loosestrife will grow well near water or in a moist part of the garden.

flower tea is a gentle sedative. An ointment can be made from the plant for treating skin complaints and stiff joints. The primulas are a group of plants which may cause skin eruptions when handled by those unfortunate enough to be allergic to them.

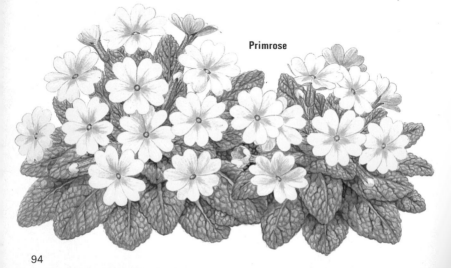

Primrose

94

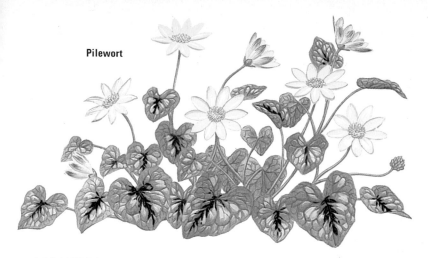

Pilewort

LOOSESTRIFE, YELLOW
Lysimachia punctata
A scentless hardy perennial with creeping rhizomes, erect downy stems (to 90cm) and broad ovate leaves, downy on the undersides. The buttercup-yellow flowers come from the axils of the leaves in pairs or small clusters, the whole forming dense terminal panicles. The wild yellow loosestrife *(L. vulgaris)* is similar but a less bushy plant.
Cultivation: by division of root. Any short piece of rhizome will make a new plant. Loosestrife does best in moist conditions beside ponds or brooks, and will spread rapidly, but if grown as a herbaceous plant it can be invasive and should be kept to its alloted area. Its robust leaf growth and bright rich yellow flowers usually attract attention and it remains in bloom for several weeks from midsummer. Having it in the garden may attract a particular bee, *Macropsis labiata*, that only visits the flower of yellow loosestrife.
Uses: at one time the herb was thought to have magic properties capable of calming disturbed animals and bringing fights between animals to an end. Hanging bunches of loosestrife under the collars or around the bodies of oxen who worked the land calmed them and made them settle to their work – it had to be magic! In fact, loosestrife repels insects and gnats and when these pests stopped tormenting the animals they would 'loose strife'! It has also been used as a vulnerary, as an infusion to bathe sore eyes and as a gargle.

Family Ranunculaceae

PILEWORT
(Lesser Celandine)
Ranunculus ficaria
A perennial with glossy leaves and shiny star-like flowers in spring. By early summer its display is over, the leaves and flowers die and it disappears until the following spring. The underground bunches of small tubers resemble immature figs, hence the specific name *ficaria* from *ficus* a fig. The dark green leaves are cordate and grow singly on erect or semi-prostrate stems (to 20–30cm). The solitary golden-yellow flowers usually have 8 petals, which fade to white at the base.
Cultivation: this cheerful little herb will give colour under trees or in shady places in spring. The tubers are dug in autumn and set where they can naturalize.
Uses: the herb, as its common name suggests, has proved an important and successful treatment for the troublesome complaint of piles (haemorrhoids). It is best used as an ointment (several members of the ranunculus family are poisonous and should not be taken internally).

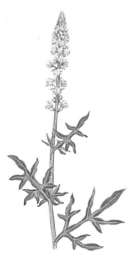

Mignonette

Family Resedaceae

MIGNONETTE
Reseda odorata
A hardy annual at first forming a rosette of lanceolate leaves and then developing square stems with alternate leaves. The spikes of tiny flowers which bloom in summer have conspicuous orange stamens which almost obscure the white petals. The whole plant has a rather sprawling habit and grows to 30–40cm.
Cultivation: from seed sown in spring in the place where it is to flower. It will grow in most soils but should not be overcrowded by other plants.
Uses: the glorious scent of this rather insignificant-looking herb is the main reason for growing it. The ancient Egyptians cherished it for its perfume and buried wreaths of mignonette with their dead. Its specific name comes from the Latin *resedo*, to appease or soothe, and it was thought to be a sedative and have healing properties. During • the 16th century it was a popular pot plant in France, favoured by the Empress Josephine for its scent. The fashion spread to England and in the 19th century it was said that 'all London smelled of Mignonette', as France was said to smell of coffee. For a time mignonette went out of favour, probably because it was not showy enough, but nostalgia for the old well-loved scented herbs and plants has brought them back into present day garden planning. In France the plant is grown commercially for its oil which is used in perfumery. The wild mignonette *(R. lutea)* is a smaller plant (to 30cm) with deeply cut leaflets and practically scentless yellowish-green flowers. Weld *(R. luteola)* grows as an erect spike (60–90cm) with entire linear leaves. It has been an important dye plant since prehistoric times and gives a range of good yellows according to the mordants and materials used. Its juice was used in the preparation of the artist's colour, Dutch pink.

Family Rosaceae

AGRIMONY
(Church Steeples, Cocklebur)
Agrimonia eupatoria
An erect downy perennial with reddish hairy stems (to 80cm). It has serrated lanceolate pinnate leaves and leaflets, the undersides greyish with soft hairs. Its slender tapering flower stalks (from which come the common name of Church Steeples) have many deep yellow 5-petalled flowers (5–10cm) opening first from the base of the spike, from midsummer. The fruit capsules, at first green then turning to tan colour, have hooked bristles which attach themselves to anything touching them, hence the name Cocklebur.
Cultivation: by seed or division of root. Self-seeds freely and will grow on most soils in a sunny position.
Uses: at one time a common roadside herb, less plentiful now as verges are often sprayed or cut before plants can seed down. Agrimony was taken as a good spring tonic, as a tea for cystitis and, externally, used to bathe sores and

wounds. A natural antibiotic which soothes inflammation, it is an effective sore throat gargle. It was an important ingredient of the famous *eau de arquebusade*, a lotion originally made from herbs to treat those injured by an arquebus or musket. Gerard claims that 'a decoction of the leaves is good for them that have naughty livers'. It is one of those wholesome herbs that may be safely taken for pleasure and will almost certainly be beneficial. Herb teas, or tisanes, are becoming more popular and a tea made from agrimony has a delicate apricot-like flavour. The herb will produce a good yellow dye.

SALAD BURNET
Sanguisorba minor (Poterium sanguisorba)
A short-lived perennial with first a rosette of round to ovate, serrated pinnate leaflets, developing branching reddish stems (to 35cm) with leaves arranged alternately. The panicles of flowers are in small round heads of florets, with protruding red-brown stamens for wind pollination. The plant has a pleasing daintiness which will appeal to flower arrangers.
Cultivation: by seed or carefully dividing the root in spring. It will grow in most soils. After flowering the stems should be cut back unless they have already been harvested for drying or are needed to ripen seed. Fresh leaf growth will emerge and survives most winters.
Uses: wild burnet, usually browsed by sheep on cliffs or downland, has a refreshing smell of cucumber when trodden on. This flavour, which seems to be combined with that of hazelnuts, makes the tender leaves an attractive addition to salads and imparts a cool flavour to summer drinks, fruit cups and punch. It can be used, fresh or dried, in wine making. It is another styptic herb which will arrest bleeding, and because of its astringency can be taken as an infusion for diarrhoea and to treat piles. Great or Garden Burnet *(Sanguisorba officinalis)*, a bigger plant (to 60cm) with longer oval flowerheads, was used medicinally in the same way. Both are decorative garden plants.

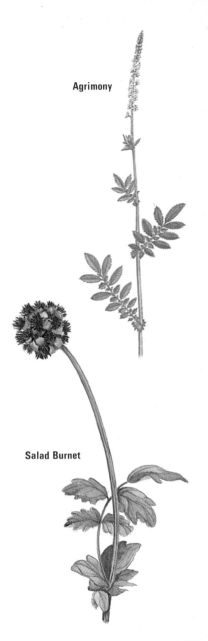

Agrimony

Salad Burnet

HERB BENNET
(Avens)
Geum urbanum

A fibrous rooted perennial with a prostrate basal growth of pinnate leaves graduating from small round pairs through ovate to a larger terminal 3-lobed leaflet which is serrated and hairy. All summer the flower stems (to 60cm), which branch at the leaf axils, have small yellow 5-petalled blooms in star-like formation with 5 long sepals and 5 short ones. The seed head of hooked achenes is more conspicuous than the flowers and, like agrimony, disperses itself by clinging to clothing and animal coats.

Cultivation: the roots may be teased apart for replanting and it will grow easily from seed. When established it self-sows freely and is best in a wild part of the garden or as ground cover under trees.

Uses: this plant has been given many names in the past, including 'clove root' and 'goldy star' (describing the scent of the root and the shape of the flower).

Some books suggest that 'the fleshy rhizomes' should be sliced and dried for flavouring, but in the present author's experience there is a great deal of fibrous root and very little rhizome one could describe as fleshy. However if the thicker of the fibrous roots are cut out, washed and dried slowly and carefully, a pleasant clove-like aroma emerges. The dried roots should be stored in airtight containers and ground when required. Towards the end of March, or as soon as the soil dries out a little, is the time when the roots are most fragrant. Herb bennet was once thought to be a Blessed Herb and was worn as an amulet or somewhere about the person to give protection from evil spirits. An infusion can be taken as a bitter tonic or used to bathe inflamed areas or sore places. It was one of the herbs used in ale making and may be of interest to home brewers.

LADY'S MANTLE
Alchemilla vulgaris

A low-growing perennial (to 30cm) with beautiful palmate, pleated leaves which are hairy at the edges. The stem leaves are smaller than those growing from the rootstock and the plant is sprawling in habit. The tiny pale lime green flowers have no petals and are on branching cymes. *Alchemilla conjuncta sericea* is similar in size and particularly attractive because the undersides of the

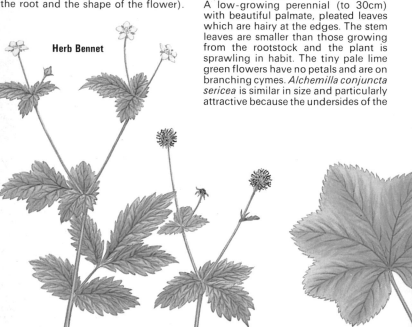

Herb Bennet

leaves are covered with silky hairs, giving them a pretty silvered look. *A. mollis* is a larger ornamental plant (to 60cm) with effective dense cymes of yellow-green petal-less flowers in summer which are cherished by flower arrangers. There are other cultivars.

Cultivation: by seed or division of root in spring or autumn. It does well in most soils and situations.

Uses: the name *alchemilla* is derived from alchemy or magic; the dew collected in the folds of the leaves was used in magic potions, and was thought to bestow beauty on those who bathed their faces with it. There is certainly magic in the beauty of the plants themselves when the sun catches raindrops or dew drops adhering to the edges of the leaves, or when the flowers fall in a frothy mass over a sun-baked old brick wall. Medicinally, alchemillas play a useful role as astringent and styptic herbs to treat diarrhoea and bleeding.

Meadowsweet

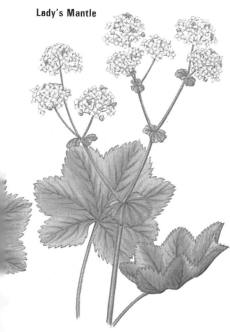

Lady's Mantle

MEADOWSWEET
(Queen of the meadow)
Filipendula ulmaria

A hardy perennial with a thick rootstock from which reddish stems grow up to 100cm. The pinnate, ovate, toothed leaves are downy on the undersides and arranged alternately in two large and two small pairs. The dense corymbs of tiny creamy flowers are sweetly scented from early summer and the leaves are subtly fragrant.

Cultivation: from division of root in spring or autumn. A moisture-loving plant, meadowsweet will thrive on heavy soils.

Uses: meadowsweet contains salicylic acid from which aspirin (the word comes from *spiraea*) was first derived. Nowadays aspirin is produced synthetically but meadowsweet is still taken as an infusion for rheumatic and arthritic complaints and as a pleasant and gentle sedative. A tea made from flowers of meadowsweet and elder is good to take at the onset of a cold or feverish condition, so it is worth drying the flowers for winter use. The flowers and leaves can be used in salads and soups.

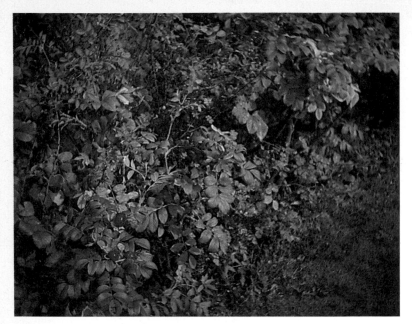

Rosehips provide one of the richest sources of vitamin C, abundant in the round, tomato-like fruits of R. rugosa.

SWEETBRIAR ROSE
(Eglantine)
Rosa rubiginosa (R. eglanteria)
A hardy shrub rose with branching stems (to 2m). The scented leaves have 5–7 ovate leaflets, and the single flowers of pale or blush pink in summer are followed by red hips in autumn.

Cultivation: from seed in spring or cuttings taken in late summer or autumn. The wild sweetbriar is the parent of many hybrids of different colours, among them the Penzance briars: Lady Penzance (copper), Julia Mannering (pale pink), Amy Robsart (deep rose pink) and Meg Merrilees (crimson). All can be trimmed as scented hedging plants, but if there is room the bushes should be allowed to grow naturally among other shrubs. If planted in different parts of the garden their apple-scented fragrance will give delight, especially after a shower of rain or in the cool of summer evenings. The scent is evident from the first breaking of the leaf buds in spring until they fall in autumn, whether the plant is in flower or not. As the bushes grow, cut out dead wood and after a few years cut them back to allow new growth.

Uses: the young leaf buds and flower petals can be added to salads and the hips used for wine or rosehip syrup.

WILD STRAWBERRY
Fragaria vesca
A low-growing hairy perennial on woody rootstock from which runners spread and form new roots. The leaf consists of three pointed, ovate leaflets with serrated edges and a long terminal point. They are strongly veined and shiny on the surface; the undersides paler with hairs. The flowers, borne on upright stems, have 5 broad white petals, and there are small round fragrant fruits.

Cultivation: by detaching runners and planting in good compost to encourage strong roots. Varieties of alpine strawberries can be obtained from many nurseries and will spread and naturalize in a position which gets a little shade as well as sun.

Uses: the fruits contain vitamin C and are good in fruit salads and summer drinks and give a special flavour to jam made from cultivated strawberries. An infusion of the leaves and flowers makes a refreshing tisane which, when cooled, may be used to bathe the face on hot summer days.

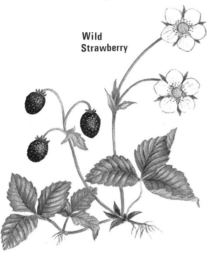

Wild Strawberry

Family Rutaceae

RUE
(Herb of grace)
Ruta graveolens
A bushy perennial with woody stems and alternate blue-green leaves with deeply divided leaflets. The yellow flowers have 4 separated petals and prominent stamens. The cultivar, Jackman's Blue rue, has denser spatulate foliage of deep blue-green.

Cultivation: by seed or cuttings in spring. Jackman's Blue rue is best propagated from cuttings to ensure that it comes true. Well-drained soil and a position where the plants get some shade in the heat of the day seems to suit them best.

Uses: for hundreds of years this herb was used in the treatment of disease and bunches were carried to give protection from pestilence. It was an ingredient of the Vinegar of the Four Thieves (see garlic) and of an infamous medication known as Gilbert's Puppy Dog Ointment concocted by an Englishman, Gilbertus Anglicus, in the 15th century: 'Take a very fat puppy dog and skin him; then take the juice of cucumber, rue and pellitory; berries of ivy and juniper; fat of vulture, fox, goose and bear in equal parts; stuff the puppy therewith and boil him; add wax to the grease that floats on the surface and make therefrom an ointment.' Rue water was sprinkled to rid houses of fleas and the sprigs of the herb were used to sprinkle holy water before Mass, hence Shakespeare's reference in 'Hamlet' to the 'herb of grace o' Sundays'. Rue has a strange smell which, with better acquaintance, becomes intriguing rather than unpleasant. A leaf or so may be added to salads and a weak infusion can be drunk as a digestive, but the beauty of its foliage alone is sufficient reason to grow rue. It is said that sage and rue will not flourish if planted near each other, but long experience of growing them in close proximity has not confirmed this. However, as there seems to be an affinity between some plants, there may also be an intolerance. Rue, like primulas and chrysanthemums, can cause skin troubles in those allergic to it.

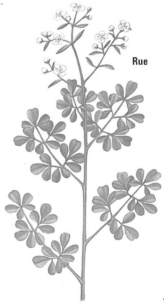

Rue

Family Scrophulariaceae

EYEBRIGHT
(Euphrasy)
Euphrasia rostkoviana (E. officinalis)
A small erect branching annual (to 30cm) with ovate, sharply-serrated leaves in opposite pairs. The inflorescence comprises short spikes of pale mauve-white flowers with two purple-veined lips, the larger lower one with three cleft lobes and a yellow spot at the throat. There are glandular hairs on the calyx. Eyebright, which grows wild on downs and heaths, is semi-parasitic on some species of grass so is not easy to establish in cultivation. It is a variable plant and there is some controversy over its classification, but it is only considered a medicinal herb if the glandular hairs are present on the calyx.

Uses: the markings of the flower may once have suggested bloodshot eyes and its main use in herbal medicine is still in opthalmic treatments. Milton brings the use of eyebright into his poetry, giving it early fame by writing of the Archangel Michael removing the film from Adam's eyes with euphrasia and rue after his fall from grace in the garden of Eden 'for he had much to see'. In many parts of the world it is regarded as a specific cure for inflammation of the eyes. Owing to the problem of cultivating it as one would other herbs in the garden, cooled and carefully-strained infusions of loosestrife, fennel or comfrey can be substituted to bathe sore eyes.

FIGWORT
(Knotted Figwort)
Scrophularia nodosa
A hardy perennial on roots of knotted thickened rhizomes, with erect square stems (to 100cm). The basal leaves are ovate, the stem leaves more cordate, toothed and in opposite pairs. Inconspicuous two-lipped dull red-brown flowers are arranged in irregular cymes. They bloom from midsummer and are pollinated by wasps.

Cultivation: by seed sown in spring or autumn or by the separation of the rhizomes. Will grow in most soils and situations but its natural habitat is a moist semi-shady situation.

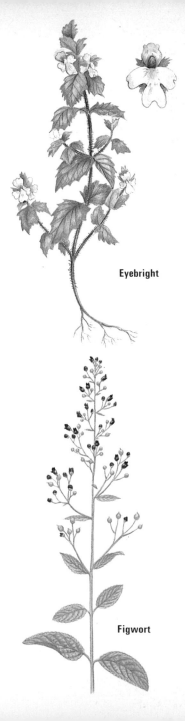

Eyebright

Figwort

102

Uses: Figwort is an interesting but unspectacular-looking plant with a long history of medicinal usage for a variety of ills such as skin problems, piles, burns and ulcers and as a liver tonic. Some of its constituents, however, are not yet fully understood nor their potential assessed, so it is best to restrict its home use to external dressings for swellings, sprains, skin rashes and the treatment of haemorrhoids. Its common name of Carpenter's Herb could have been earned by its providing first aid to stop bleeding from accidents with tools, or simply because its long tough straight square stems were used as measuring rods. In France it is called *Herbe du siège* as its tuberous roots provided famine food during a siege by Richelieu's army in 1628. It is unappetising and not to be recommended for culinary use, but it was held in great esteem in the past.

GREAT MULLEIN
(Beggar's Blanket)
Verbascum thapsus
A stout biennial (to 100–130cm). From the taproot in the first year grows a flat rosette of downy flannel-like leaves (30cm or more in length), entire, ovate-lanceolate. In the second year the leaves diminish in size as they ascend the stems. The stems, sometimes branching, terminate in dense spikes of yellow flowers with 5 flattened petal-like lobes joined at the base of the corolla which are out of character with the two-lipped flowers of this family.
Cultivation: by seed sown in autumn or spring. It will grow in most reasonably well-drained soils and is usually found growing wild on waste ground and dry hedge banks. There are several wild species differing in size and shade of flower colour, but all with more or less woolly leaves.
Uses: great mullein has over thirty common names (candlewick plant, hag's taper, feltwort and many more) all suggesting uses to which this herb has been put. The names beggar's blanket and old man's flannel suggest the warmth the large downy leaves would give to chilly bones when tucked inside thin garments. Feltwort describes the felt-like texture of the leaves. Their

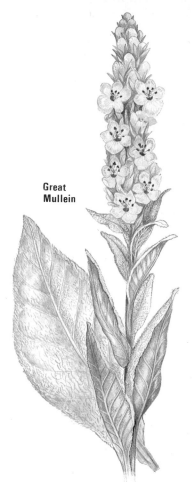

Great
Mullein

woolly surface used to be rolled off and used as a wick for lights, while the whole spike was dipped in tallow and carried as a torch. The flowers are used as an infusion or made into a syrup with honey for all chest complaints. When dried, the leaves and flowers can be combined with herbs like coltsfoot and clover to make a herbal smoking mixture for bronchial troubles. The emollient properties of the herb can be made use of in poultices and fomentations, and a yellow dye is made from the flowers.

Family Tropaeolaceae

NASTURTIUM
Tropaeolum majus
An annual herb with entire round leaves
(5–10cm), a little wavy at the edges,
growing on brittle pale green leaf stalks.
The spurred flowers (5–7cm) vary in
colour from pale yellow to bronze and
shades of red.
Cultivation: the large seeds are sown
in spring spaced 10–20cm apart and
pushed 3cm into the soil. Nasturtium
thrives happily in a sunny place but will
give a welcome patch of colour in semi-
shade. A richly-coloured variety which
holds its flowers well up above the
leaves is Cherry Rose.
Uses: in addition to its ornamental
interest as a bush plant, trailer or
climber it is a salad herb which may be
used in place of watercress *(Nasturtium
officinale)*. It gets its name from the hot
cress flavour which has a tendency to
act as a 'nasturtium' or nose twister!
The green unripe seeds can be soaked
in salted water for 12 hours, rinsed in
fresh water and then packed into
bottles with spiced or dill vinegar
poured over them. They are used
instead of capers, but will taste better if
kept for 6 months first. The leaves
contain vitamin C and have a natural
antibiotic action.

Family Umbelliferae

ANGELICA
Angelica Archangelica
Although botanically classified as a
biennial this herb may live for several
years. On thick branching roots it
makes substantial growth the first year
into a clump of hollow stems with light
green leaves, subdivided into leaflets
with serrated edges. In the second year
the central flower stem grows up to
100–150cm, carrying rounded umbels
of tiny yellow-green florets, followed
by masses of flattened oval seeds.
Cultivation: the viable life of angelica
seed is short and they should be sown
in autumn when fully ripe and not kept
until spring. The young seedlings will
lose their leaves for the winter (as the
parent plant also dies down) but they
reappear in spring, usually in large
quantities. This big plant needs adequate moisture in the soil to maintain
its growth and does well in a heavy soil.
Angelica flourishes in Lapland and the
Scandinavian countries so there is little
doubt about its hardiness for garden
cultivation. In the past it was regarded
as an important medicinal herb; legend
tells that it acquired the distinctive title
of Archangelica because the Archangel
Michael appeared in a dream to a monk
in time of plague, instructing the people

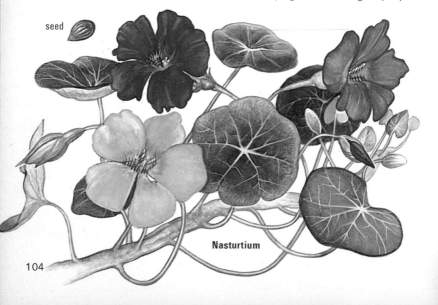

seed

Nasturtium

to chew angelica root as a protective measure. It is used in the treatment of bronchitis and to stimulate appetite in those debilitated by illness. A pleasant after-dinner tisane made from the leaves acts as a carminative. The stalks give interesting results when blended with rhubarb, gooseberry or marrow for jams and conserves, or when making elderflower wine. It is an ingredient of vermouth, Benedictine and other liqueurs. The candied stalks are familiar as cake and dessert decoration. Home-candied angelica is delicious and, although the process is spread over a couple of days, it is very simple to make. Using only the tender basal stalks towards the end of May, cut them into 10cm lengths, put in a pan with just enough water to cover them and boil gently until soft. Drain and strip off the fine outer skin. Weigh the stalks and add the same amount of sugar and leave in a covered bowl (not metal) for two days. They will have made syrup by this time and should be brought to the boil and simmered gently until the angelica clears. A drop of good green colouring may be added if liked. Drain through a colander, dip the sticks in icing sugar and put on a cake rack in a cool oven to dry off; but do not allow them to get too hard. Store between layers of greaseproof paper in airtight boxes.

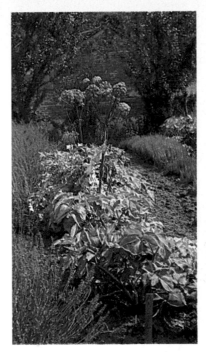

Angelica has a striking head of flowers. The stalks at the base of the plant are used for candying.

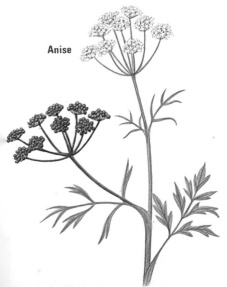

Anise

ANISE
Pimpinella anisum

A tender half-hardy annual (to 50cm) with a thin taproot and erect stems bearing broad, deeply-lobed and toothed leaves at the base and finely cut narrow leaflets up the stem. Branching flower stems terminate in compound umbels of tiny white or cream flowers, followed by ribbed seeds, brown when ripe.

Cultivation: by seed sown in early summer outside or a little earlier in pots indoors for protection if the weather is poor.

Uses: the warm aromatic flavour of aniseed is familiar to most people. An excellent digestive, the seeds can be chewed after a meal or a tisane made from seeds or leaves. It can be used instead of fennel to dress fish, with egg dishes and in salads.

CARAWAY
Carum carvi

A biennial with a slender taproot and erect stems (to 50cm), the leaves consisting of many finely cut leaflets. The flowers are in compound umbels of tiny white florets followed by narrow ridged green seeds ($\frac{1}{2}$cm) which are brown when ripe.

Cultivation: from seed sown in early autumn the young plants overwinter and come into flower late the following spring, ripening seed in early summer. The plant dies after seeding but on light soil will self-sow and continue the cycle. A light well-drained soil and sunny position is advised but caraway will succeed on well-worked heavy soil.

Uses: for 5000 years or so this herb has acted as a carminative and cured digestive troubles in children and adults. It is the flavouring agent of the liqueur Kummel and is used in cheeses, cakes, breads, biscuits, with fruit dishes and vegetables. Those who dislike the

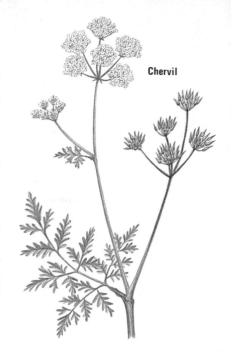

Chervil

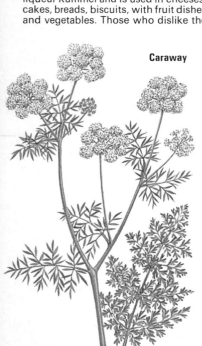

Caraway

grittiness of caraway seeds in cakes and buns may like to try using the seeds when they are green and succulent, at which time they impart their flavour but are not hard. The roots, grated raw in salads or cooked like small parsnips as a vegetable, are good served with pork. The leaves can be used for salads and soups. In the past caraway was recommended for 'pale faced girls', perhaps because it stimulated their appetites and so made them look rosier, and it was put into love potions to encourage faithfulness. Pigeon fanciers will know that their birds do not stray if caraway is added to their food.

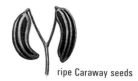

ripe Caraway seeds

CHERVIL
Anthriscus cerefolium
An attractive fragrant biennial (to 30c) with deeply cut ferny leaves consisting of pinnate and terminal leaflets. It has umbels of tiny white flowers and thin seeds ($\frac{1}{2}$–1cm).

Cultivation: seed is best sown in late summer when it ripens on the plant; the young seedlings will overwinter and grow on in spring. If it is to be dried it should be cut as soon as it is big enough to prevent it flowering and seeding; dry weather accelerates this maturing process. The leaves are sometimes tinged with pink, but for drying only the green ones are taken.

Uses: this pretty plant with lacy foliage is ornamental to grow and the slightly accented anise-flavoured leaves are delicious in salads, with fish, egg and cheese dishes, in sauces, savoury dips and as a garnish on soups. Its flavour is lost in long cooking so it should be used fresh and added at the last moment. It freezes well and makes an interesting alternative to parsley. Grown in a pot on the kitchen window sill it will provide fresh snippets of flavour during the winter.

CORIANDER
Coriandrum sativum
An annual (50–60cm) with erect, branching stems, deeply cut broadly segmented lower leaves and finely feathery upper stem leaves. The pale pink flowers are in light umbels and mature as small round ridged green fruits, biscuit-coloured when ripe.

Cultivation: by seed sown as soon as the soil is workable in spring. Covering them with a cloche in their early stages will be helpful. Coriander is fairly hardy and will grow on most soils that are in good condition, but a sunny situation is needed to ripen the seeds.

Uses: the flavour of home-grown coriander is superb and it improves as the seeds are stored, which must be when totally dry and in airtight containers. Coriander is an ancient herb widely used in cooking. It is a basic flavouring for curries and is used in chutneys and pickles, with yoghourts and dips, fruit and vegetables. If fresh

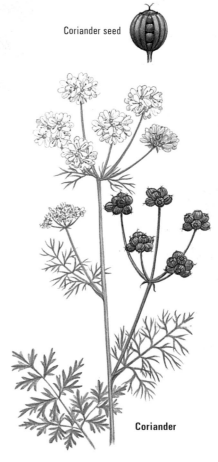

Coriander seed

Coriander

leaves are wanted, some plants should be discouraged from flowering by cutting out the potential flower stalks to stimulate more leaf growth. The leaves are used in curries and chutneys to serve with curry. The disagreeable smell so often mentioned in connection with coriander leaves and green seeds is not always apparent and certainly need not be a deterrent to using this aromatic herb. It will often be found that the seeds that ripen on the plants are bigger than those sown from the seed packet.

CUMIN

Cuminum cyminum

An annual with a thin taproot, branching slender stems (15–20cm) and fine thread-like foliage. The irregular umbels of small pinkish-white flowers mature to ridged seeds similar to those of caraway.

Cultivation: sow seed indoors in pots or boxes in spring. In late May or June if the weather is suitable, carefully transplant to a warm, sheltered place. Keep a ball of compost around the plants so as not to disturb the roots. It may be wise to keep some plants in pots so that they can be protected if the weather is unfavourable to this tender herb.

Uses: this is another herb which has been in use for thousands of years as a carminative. The seeds give a warm pungency to curries and stews and are used with courgettes and marrows, in herb vinegars and as a tisane to aid digestion after meals.

DILL

Anethum graveolens

A hardy annual (to 90cm) with hollow erect stems and feathery leaves which have finely cut thread-like leaflets of a bluish-green. The inflorescence is a dainty rounded compound umbel of many clusters of tiny yellow florets.

Cultivation: from seed sown in spring where it is to grow because, like most of the other annual umbellifers, it does not transplant well. It will grow in most soils but likes a sunny site.

Uses: though similar in appearance dill and fennel have quite different scents and flavours and if the liquorice taste of fennel is not liked, dill may be found pleasant as an alternative. It is a popular herb in Scandinavian countries, the Norse word *dilla* means to lull. Dill water, a simple infusion of the leaves or seeds, is used to soothe babies with wind or stomach upsets. Use freshly chopped with new potatoes, peas, fish, omelettes, salads and pickles.

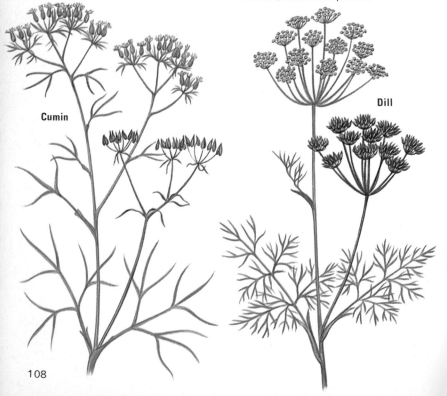

Cumin

Dill

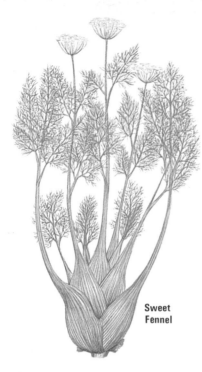

Sweet Fennel

FENNEL
Foeniculum vulgare (F. officinalis)
A tall hardy perennial with a thick tap-root and hollow stems (100–150cm). The feathery leaves are formed of bright green thread-like leaflets. The flower is a flat umbel of tiny yellow florets.

Cultivation: by seed sown in spring or autumn. This herb will grow in most soils in an open situation and self-sows freely on light soils.

Uses: in spring the tender young stalks can be peeled of their outer skin (like rhubarb) and eaten raw like celery or used in salads. Sprays of fennel leaves cooked with fish are best removed before serving and fresh ones used as a garnish, or in a sauce served with the dish. Fennel is 'a gallant expeller of the wind' and at one time was thought to be a slimming herb, possibly because eating it is alleged to take away the pangs of hunger. It is also said to be most soothing when used to bathe sore eyes. Bronze fennel *(F. vulgare pur-*

purea) is similar in habit to the green-leaved type, but it is of particular interest for the beauty of its deep bronze-coloured foliage. It is an ornamental plant to grow and cut for foliage arrangements but it can also be used for the same culinary and medicinal purposes as green fennel. Sweet or Florence fennel *(F. dulce)* is the annual variety which produces the swollen stem bases which look rather like celery. The perennial fennels will not do so. The plant grows to about 60cm and should be carefully cultivated as a kitchen garden vegetable, the seedlings being thinned to 10cm. Home-grown plants do not usually reach the size of those imported from the continent, but the flavour is good and they can be freshly cut and eaten raw as a salad herb or cooked and served with oil, butter or a sauce. If fennel leaf is to be dried or frozen, sweet fennel is excellent as it makes abundant leaf growth which may be cut frequently and renews quickly.

The feathery foliage of bronze fennel is particularly beautiful in spring.

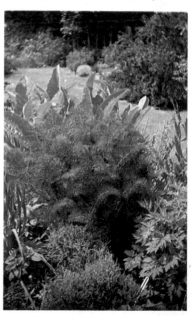

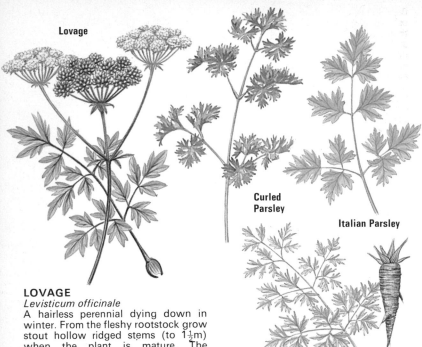

Lovage

Curled Parsley

Italian Parsley

Hamburg Parsley

LOVAGE
Levisticum officinale

A hairless perennial dying down in winter. From the fleshy rootstock grow stout hollow ridged stems (to 1½m) when the plant is mature. The yellowish-green leaves consist of 3 serrated ovate or deeply indented leaflets and the small yellow flowers which appear in late summer are in terminal compound umbels.

Cultivation: from seed in early autumn or late spring. The roots can be cut to give a piece of root with a bud or 'eye' attached and replanted in spring. The plant needs a good deep soil which will not dry out in summer.

Uses: when the first shoots emerge in spring with bronze-green foliage it is worth covering them with an inverted bucket to 'force' them for early salads. The celery flavour is welcome in many contexts – once acquainted with lovage it will probably become a favourite herb. The herb dries well and will give flavour to soups and stews in winter. If the plant is to be dried it is well to cut out the flowering stalks to promote more leafy growth. The tender young stalks can be eaten like sticks of celery. Lovage aids digestion, acts as a mild diuretic and may be helpful to sufferers from rheumatism.

PARSLEY
(Moss curled parsley)
Petroselinum crispum

A biennial on a short taproot with deeply divided leaflets which form the familiar curly rich green foliage. If allowed to flower the ridged stalks produce umbels of pale yellowish-green tiny florets.

Cultivation and uses: sow seed in late summer or spring. Parsley needs a good moisture-retaining soil and will do well in partial shade as well as full sunlight. The flower stalks should be removed to prolong leaf production. Many theories exist as to the quickest way to get parsley to germinate, as it can take as long as 6–8 weeks if sown on dry soil. It is said that it goes to the Devil 7 times before it can grow and that it should be sown on Good Friday. In the 16th century, the gardener-herbalist Thomas Hyll wrote: 'To make the seeds appear more quickly, steep them in vinegar and strew the bed with ashes of beanwater and best aqua vitae, then cover the bed with a woollen cloth and the plants will begin to appear in an hour. Then take off the cloth that they may shoot up higher to the wonder of all beholders.' Less dramatic, saving the brandy for better uses and without the mysterious 'ashes of beanwater', have ready a piece of black polythene the size of the proposed parsley bed, which should be raked to a fine tilth; soak the seeds overnight in vinegar and next day sow them on the surface of the soil, tamping them in with the back of a rake. Cover with the polythene, pulling soil up over all the edges to make a seal and prevent it moving. Leave for 8 days and then lift a corner every day to see whether a flush of seedlings is visible. As soon as they appear, remove the cover, keep watered if the weather is dry and let the parsley grow on naturally. It is worth waiting for moist warm conditions ('growing weather') to start a parsley bed. To grow it indoors, make a parsley ball. Shape fine mesh chicken wire into a hollow ball, line it with moss and fill with good compost. Carefully pass enough young parsley roots through the wire, leaving 5–8cm between them. Top up with compost, close the top of the 'ball', water well and hang in a kitchen window. In time the whole ball should be a curly mass of foliage. Plain-leaved Italian parsley *(P. hortense filicinum)* has flat deeply indented trifoliate leaves and a strong flavour, and Hamburg Parsley *(P. sativum tuberosum)* which grows like a parsnip or sometimes like a turnip, may be grated raw for salads or cooked as a vegetable. All are grown from seed. Parsley, familiar as a garnish and flavouring for stuffings, soups and sauces, stimulates the appetite and acts as a diuretic. Eaten after garlic, it helps to destroy the odour.

SWEET CICELY
Myrrhis odorata
A hardy perennial dying down in winter. From the large rootstock buds develop into hollow, branching stems (to 95cm) with bright green hairy, deeply segmented pinnate leaflets, some with white blotches. The tiny white flowers are in compound umbels (5–10cm across).

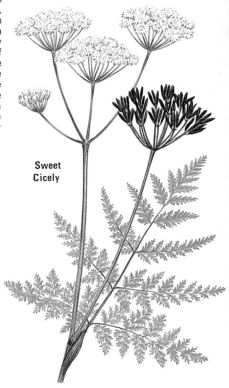

Sweet Cicely

Cultivation: by division of root crown or seed sown in late autumn and left to stratify in the cold soil of winter and germinate in spring. The plant likes a moisture-retaining soil but with adequate humus will flourish in most soils.

Uses: all parts of the plant are anise-flavoured and sweet to taste. The young stems can be peeled and eaten. Leaves and stems added to early gooseberries, rhubarb or later to plums which may not be fully ripe, will take away the tartness of the fruit and less sugar can be used in cooking them. Sweet cicely is used by diabetics as a sugar substitute. The true anise flavour of this perennial herb is a good alternative to the tender annual anise. Also called Greater Chervil, it can be used instead of the biennial chervil.

Family Urticaceae

NETTLE
Urtica dioica

A persistent perennial growing over 1 m in height from creeping rootstock, with erect stems bearing opposite and alternate pairs of sharply serrated heart-shaped leaves which are hairy and stinging. Male and female flowers are on different plants and the infloresence, coming from the axils of the leaves,

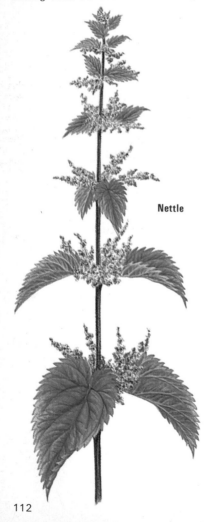

Nettle

hangs as drooping racemes of small greenish florets without petals, which are wind pollinated.

Cultivation and uses: any pieces of rhizome pulled off and replanted will quickly establish. Nettle is not a herb usually encouraged in cultivation – the effort is rather to eradicate it – but in a wild area there are reasons for letting it flourish. Probably one of the most underestimated growing herbs, it is an invaluable plant which has been a source of food, medicine, fibre and dyes since the Bronze Age. Among its known constituents are iron, calcium, potassium and other trace elements, vitamins A and C, and histamine. It has a wide application for treating internal and external bleeding, haemorrhoids, and many skin complaints, including eczema and urticaria (nettle rash). It can lower the blood sugar level and is used in the treatment of rheumatism. In the past it was a vital spring green vegetable, helping to purify blood and clear up vitamin deficiency ailments caused by poor winter diet; while nettle tea and nettle beer were favourite spring beverages. It is richer in iron and vitamins than spinach. Cook the young leaves in the water adhering to them after they have been washed, add a little olive oil or butter, and serve with poached eggs, grated cheese, nutmeg or a squeeze of lemon juice. Combine them with leeks or watercress for soup. The plants contain natural sugar, starch and protein. When the plants are allowed to grow they become coarse and are not suitable for eating, but if cut down to ground level tender young leaves will soon come again. The mature plants were once used as an important fibre in clothmaking. It was an alternative to cotton and in some cases considered superior to flax. Nettles have also been employed in the manufacture of paper, of commercial chlorophyll, and as a dye. Cut, dried nettle is fed to poultry, goats and cattle; and the caterpillars of many butterflies – comma, small tortoiseshell, red admiral, peacock and painted lady – feed on the leaves. An infusion of nettles can be used as a feed for houseplants. The annual nettle *(Urtica urens)* is a smaller plant which has the same properties as the common stinging nettle.

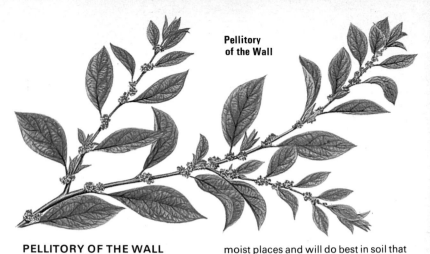

Pellitory
of the Wall

PELLITORY OF THE WALL
Parietaria diffusa (P. officinalis)
A perennial plant with fibrous roots.
The branching red stems (to 60cm) are
almost transparent, with entire, pointed
ovate mealy leaves. Clusters of red-
green flowers without petals appear in
the axils of the leaves, blooming
through summer.
Cultivation: from division of root in
spring or autumn. As its name suggests,
it grows in shallow soil.
Uses: pellitory has a reputation as an
effective treatment for cystitis and
stones in the bladder (it is best taken as
an infusion in frequent small doses). It
contains sulphur, calcium and potassium salts, and can be an irritant to
sufferers from hay fever.

Family Valerianaceae

VALERIAN
(Phu)
Valeriana officinalis
A hardy perennial with slender rhizomes radiating from the centre of the
rootstock. In spring lanceolate, pinnate
radical leaves, some toothed, form a
basal clump from which grow the
ridged, hollow, flowering stems
(90–120cm) with terminal corymbs of
pale pink tubular florets.
Cultivation: division of rootstock is
easily achieved by detaching plantlets
from the outside of the parent plant.
Valerian is found wild in ditches and

moist places and will do best in soil that
is moisture-retaining and rich in humus.
Uses: one of the oldest-known nervine
herbs, it is used as a sedative and antispasmodic in the treatment of nervous
and anxiety problems. The root is dried
and in the process emits a powerful
tom-cat smell, hence its ancient name
of 'phu'. The time of year at which the
root is dug affects its potency.

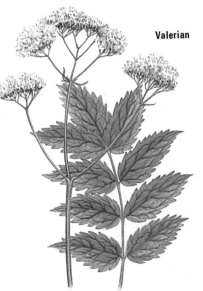

Valerian

113

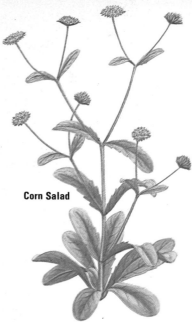

Corn Salad

Cultivation: by cuttings in late spring. Verbena should be protected in winter unless growing in temperate sheltered conditions. It looks very dead with dry pale leafless branches in winter, but in spring buds will break from the nodes.
Uses: delicious as a tea, to garnish melon and other fruits and to flavour sponge cakes. When dried, it can be put in bowls to give fragrance to a room and used as an ingredient of pot pourri.

VERVAIN
Verbena officinalis
A perennial herb with fibrous roots and a bushy growth of hairless, angular branching stems (70–90cm). The basal leaves are broad ovate, deeply indented and toothed; the stem leaves lanceolate, in opposite pairs. The two-lipped lavender-coloured flowers open from the base of a slender pointed spike.
Cultivation: from seed or division of root. This herb likes a fairly dry, sunny position and although the flowers are displayed sparsely on the spikes, their effect is dainty and elegant over many weeks in summer.
Uses: the history of vervain is confused. A herb of priests, druids and witches, it was regarded with fear in case it was used in harmful witchcraft, and with respect in the hope that it might give protection from the evil eye. It is still used as a sedative for nervous complaints and as a general tonic. It has proved beneficial in the treatment of certain skin troubles which may have been caused by nervous tension.

Family Violaceae

VIOLET
Viola odorata
A hardy perennial (to 20cm). The fibrous creeping roots spread by stolons rooting at the nodes and making new plants which, by repeating the process, soon cover the area around the original plant. The dark green heart-shaped leaves with crenate edges grow on long stalks and emit an elusive violet perfume before the flowers open. The self-fertile flowers are carried on long stems which curve over at their tips to carry a single bloom. These are commonly violet-blue but many shades exist and some flowers are double.

CORN SALAD
(Lamb's Lettuce, Loblollie)
Valerianella locusta (V. olitoria)
A hardy annual with opposite oblong leaves on much-branched stems (to 30cm). Terminal clusters of tiny pale lilac florets are found sparsely in the axils of the leaves.
Cultivation: by seed sown in succession from spring. Late summer sowing will give plants which grow on into the winter. Corn salad likes most soils and an open situation. It self-sows freely.
Uses: an easily grown salad herb of the cut-and-come-again type, best used when the leaves are young. It is hardy for winter use and was popular in the days when vegetables were scarce as a good tonic and blood cleansing food.

Family Verbenaceae

VERBENA, LEMON
Aloysia triphylla (Lippia citriodora)
A deciduous shrub (to 1m) with branching stems, lemon-scented, lanceolate leaves and slender flower spikes with pale lavender two-lipped flowers.

Cultivation: from seed or detached rooted stolons set in a humus-rich soil in a position with some shade. Because the plant propagates itself so freely it soon exhausts the ground on which it is growing and generous dressings of leafmould must be put down to prevent the soil from drying out. A violet bed benefits from being cleared of all the old plants every couple of years.

Uses: the scent and beauty of the violet have been praised by poets and writers since early classical times and there can be few people who would feel anything but pleasure in being the recipient of a bunch of violets at anytime of the year. The commercial production of violets is an important part of the flower-producing industry, and in Europe they are still grown to a limited extent for the production of violet perfume which, like lavender, remains constantly popular. The flowers were made into syrups, wines and cosmetic washes; eaten in salads, fried in oil and candied; and used medicinally for skin complaints and as poultices for ulcers.

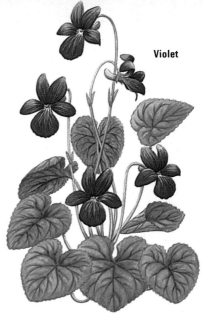

Violet

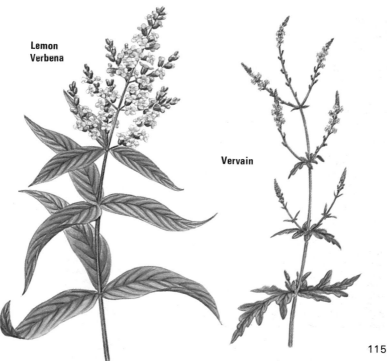

Lemon Verbena

Vervain

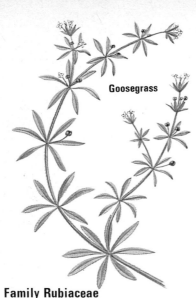

Goosegrass

Family Rubiaceae

GOOSEGRASS
(Cleavers, Everlasting Friendship)
Galium aparine
An annual which appears very early in the year and spreads rapidly. The squared stems and leaves are all furnished with hooked bristles which assist it to climb into hedges and through nearby vegetation to a length of over 1m. Groups of linear leaves and stipules are arranged in whorls at the nodes of the angular stems and tiny whitish flowers are borne on stalks springing from the axils of the leaves, ripening to round seed vessels also covered with hooked bristles. The plant 'cleaves' or clings to anything it touches – other plant material, animal fur, wool, or clothing of passers by – thus dispersing itself over a wide area.
Cultivation and uses: from seed sown in autumn when ripe, but should only be grown in a wild part of the garden. The young plant is edible; although bitter to taste, it may be chopped and eaten raw or cooked as a green vegetable. From late summer the ripe seeds can be stripped off in handfuls, roasted and ground as an alternative to coffee (the coffee shrub *Coffea arabica* from which the coffee berries of commerce are gathered,

belongs to the same natural order as goosegrass). Used as a lotion, it is considered an effective treatment for skin eruptions and taken internally as a tea can help to soothe inflammations of the bladder.

WOODRUFF
(Sweet Woodruffe)
Asperula odorata
A low-growing carpeting perennial (to 25cm) rooting on angular, erect square stems. The leaves are in whorls of 6–8 lanceolate leaflets, terminating in loose clusters of tubular, white, 4-lobed flowers.
Cultivation: by division of the slender-rooted stems in spring or autumn. It will grow best in semi-shade in a humus-rich soil and provides an attractive ground cover.
Uses: when the leaves are dried they have a delicious new-mown hay scent which comes from the coumarin released from the plant. The herb is excellent as a tisane, or used in summer fruit drinks and white wine. It has a carminative action and will help to settle an upset stomach. It makes a welcome addition to pot pourri and on its own in open bowls will give an elusive fragrance to a room.

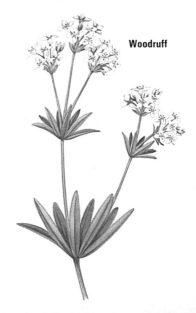

Woodruff

POISONOUS HERBS

Family Caprifoliaceae

DANEWORT
(Dwarf Elder)
Sambucus ebulus
This herbaceous perennial spreads rapidly by rhizomes. The stout ridged stems (to 100cm) bear leaves consisting of lanceolate-ovate serrated leaflets which have an unpleasant smell when bruised. The flowers are in flat cymes of pinkish-white florets from midsummer, followed by small black fruits (berries) in autumn, and the plant dies down in winter. Although its habit of growth is different to that of the shrubby elder *(Sambucus niger)*, the flowerheads and fruits can be confused, and should not be eaten as they have a very strong purgative action. The berries produce a purple dye. Danewort is an invasive plant which is difficult to eradicate.

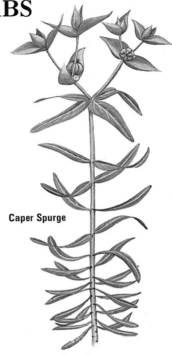

Caper Spurge

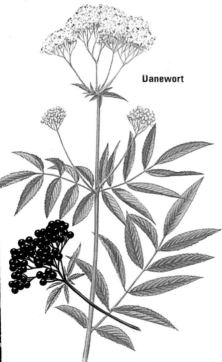

Danewort

Family Euphorbiaceae

CAPER SPURGE
Euphorbia lathyrus
A biennial with fibrous roots producing in the first year an erect stem with opposite and alternate pairs of lanceolate blue-green entire leaves (to 60cm). In the second year the terminal shoots form branching stems with pointed ovate lime-green leaves. In the axils of the leaves come inconspicuous yellowish-green flowers followed by round caper-like seed capsules and it is because of their resemblance to the flower buds of the true caper bush *(Capparis spinosa)* that this spurge gets its name. Caper spurge, which seeds freely and grows finally to 90–100cm, is of interest to flower and foliage arrangers. The caper-like fruits should not be eaten, and some people are allergic to the milky juice which runs from the stems of all spurges when cut or broken.

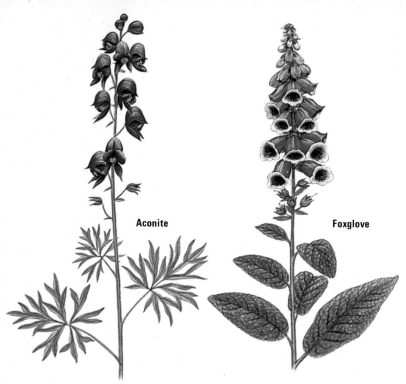

Aconite

Foxglove

Family Ranunculaceae

ACONITE
(Monkshood, Helmet Flower)
Aconitum napellus
A perennial on tuberous roots dying down in winter. The erect stems (to 1m) have dark green, shiny, deeply divided leaves. The helmet-shaped flowers of dark blue-purple are arranged as a terminal raceme. The ornamental herb grows best in semi-shade and a humus-rich soil. All parts of the plant are *extremely poisonous*; it should not be grown in gardens where young children could pick the flowers and put them, or their fingers after handling them, in their mouths. Gloves should be worn or the hands washed after dividing the roots for replanting. There are cultivars with blue and white flowers and *A. lycoctonum* (Wolfsbane) with yellow flowers. Also poisonous are the early flowering

winter aconite *(Eranthis hyemalis)* with its buttercup-yellow flowers surrounded with a green 'ruff', columbine *(Aquilegia vulgaris* and cvs.) and various buttercups *(Ranunculus sps)*.

Family Scrophulariaceae

FOXGLOVES
(Fairy thimbles, Deadmen's bells)
Digitalis purpurea
A biennial on fibrous roots with, in the first year, a rosette of wrinkled broad lanceolate or ovate leaves, softly hairy on their undersides. In the second year the familiar erect stem grows to 100cm or more, bearing one-sided racemes of purple bell flowers with darker spots on their insides. The generic name comes from the shape of the flower, which looks like a finger or digit. Foxglove plays an important role in medicine, yielding the drug digitalin which is

used for the treatment of some heart complaints. It must only be administered under medical supervision. The first year's rosette of radical leaves could be confused with early growth of comfrey, but if the backs of the leaves are drawn across the back of the hand, it will be found that the foxglove's leaves are softly hairy, while the comfrey's are rough and scratchy with coarse hairs. The root of foxglove is fibrous; that of comfrey a thick taproot. In Wales the juice from the crushed leaves was used as a colouring agent to accentuate the pattern engraved on stone floors for decoration, as earlier mud floors had designs scratched in them.

Family Solanaceae

DEADLY NIGHTSHADE
(Belladonna)
Atropa belladonna
A hardy perennial dying down in winter. From thick fleshy rootstocks the stout stems grow in spring, forming branched bushy plants (90 100cm). The dull green leaves are ovate, entire and arranged in pairs. The single, drooping drab purple flowers, bell-shaped with five lobes, come from the axils of the leaves. They are followed in autumn by a single berry about the size of a cherry, green first and then ripening to glossy black, with a prominent five-

pointed calyx beneath. This plant yields hyoscyamine and atropine, and, in professional hands, has important medical applications, but its name is no exaggeration – all parts of it are poisonous and it can be deadly if wrongly used. Children should be made aware of the dangerous nature of the attractive-looking berries. The plant acquired the name belladonna (beautiful lady) because it was used to dilate the pupils of the eyes. It is a sinister-looking plant when in flower and it is not difficult to believe the stories of it having been given as a drink to poison enemies. Woody nightshade or bitter-sweet *(S. dulcamara)* trails through hedgerows in summer, its purple flowers having 5-pointed corollas and prominent pyramids of yellow anthers, followed by green and then red berries in autumn. These are poisonous to eat, as are the fruits of the potato plant *(S. tuberosum)* which come after the flowers have faded and look rather like small green tomatoes. Care should be taken when preparing potatoes for cooking that any parts of the tubers which have turned green by being over-exposed to light are rejected, as the green part can be toxic.

The glossy black berries of deadly nightshade, like all parts of the plant, are very poisonous.

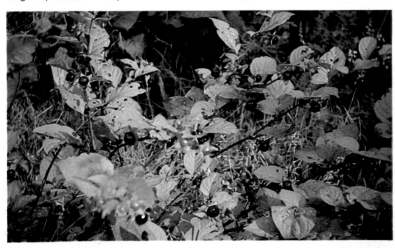

HENBANE
(Henbell)
Hyoscyamus niger
A biennial (occasionally annual) herb producing first a rosette of grey-green pointed lanceolate and coarsely toothed leaves which are hairy and sticky to the touch. These die down in winter but in spring shoots emerge to form a branching bushy plant (to 100cm). The funnel-shaped flowers with 5 lobes are of an unattractive dull cream-buff shade, heavily-veined and spotted with purple. They are arranged as one-sided spikes, and reinforce the sinister impression made by this unpleasant-smelling plant. Henbane is poisonous in every part, and although it has been used from the earliest known times as an effective, safe sedative and pain-killer, it is lethal in amateur hands and must never be taken internally. The annual variety, a smaller plant (to 60cm), is usually unbranched. It is also toxic.

THORNAPPLE
(Jimson weed)
Datura stramonium
An annual of curious and interesting appearance and unpleasant smell which is poisonous in all parts if taken internally other than under strict medical supervision. Thornapple makes a branching bushy plant (60–90cm) with broad ovate irregularly lobed leaves (10–20cm), grey-green and prominently veined. The handsome funnel-shaped white flowers (to 8cm) grow singly from the axil of a leaf or stem and open at night to emit a fragrance which attracts moths, as does the night-scented tobacco plant *(Nicotiana affinis)* of the same family. The seed capsule brings to mind the spiked

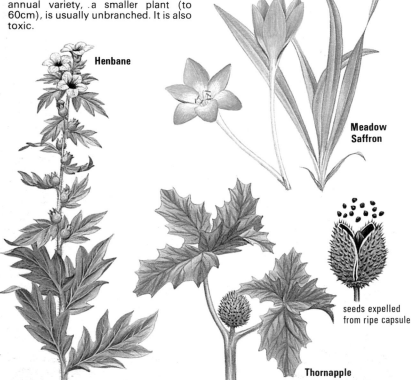

Henbane

Meadow Saffron

seeds expelled from ripe capsule

Thornapple

casing of the horse chestnut 'conker'. It is about the same size but when it splits open is found to contain a central section with many brown-black seeds. In America this plant is known as Devil's apple because of the bad effects caused by eating it. The seed remains viable over many years and is known to have reappeared in one place 18 years after it was first grown there.

Family Liliaceae

MEADOW SAFFRON
(Colchicum, Naked Ladies)
Colchicum autumnale
An attractive perennial growing from a corm and producing bright green lanceolate leaves in spring with oval fruits (to 3cm) on stalks 15–20cm long. These die down before the 'naked ladies', leafless 6-petalled rosy-purple flowers, emerge in autumn on what appear to be long white stalks but are in

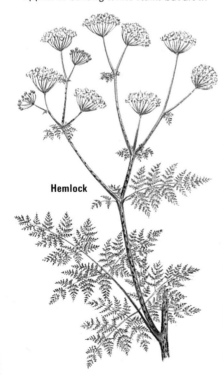

Hemlock

fact the elongated corolla tubes. The plant looks best coming up through ground cover (otherwise the bare 'stalks' look rather stark), and will give a welcome patch of colour and flourish even on heavy soil. As this herb is poisonous it must not be confused with the true saffron *Crocus sativus* (see page 51). Although saffron also flowers in autumn, the blooms are small and typically crocus-like; the leaves in spring are finely linear.

Family Umbelliferae

HEMLOCK
(Poison Parsley, Spotted Hemlock)
Conium maculatum
A biennial, growing in the second year to 150cm with erect branching stems. This is the only white-flowered umbellifer with hollow stems marked with purple spots or blotches. Many plants of this family have purple streaking on the stems, or one side of the stem may be purple and the other green, but a positive way of identifying hemlock is by the presence of the purple spots and an unpleasant stuffy, mousey smell when the leaves are bruised. The foliage is ferny, finely cut and elegant and the flowers are in terminal umbels of tiny white florets. All parts of this plant are deadly poisonous and it achieved fame long ago as the source of the poison which was administered to the learned Socrates. Many members of this family have similar ferny foliage and that of the wholesome sweet cicely is not dissimilar, but all parts of sweet cicely are easily identified by the strong smell of anise when the plant is crushed. Lesser hemlock or fool's parsley *(Aethusa cynapium)* is a small annual umbellifer (to 25cm) with flat pinnate leaflets similar to the plain-leaved parsley but distinguished by pointed slender bracts underneath the umbels of white flowers, giving the head a bearded appearance. Hemlock water dropwort *(Oenanthe crocata)* is a hairless perennial (to 100cm) with hollow stems, shiny broad indented leaflets and dense umbels of white florets. As the name suggests, the plant is found near water and should not be eaten although the leaves smell deceptively of parsley.

GLOSSARY

achene: a small nut-like fruit; a carpel containing a single seed.

antispasmodic: relieves convulsive or spasmodic pains.

antiviral: a substance capable of attacking some virus infections.

axil: the angle between the stem and the upper side of the leaf stalk.

bract: modified leaf-like structure.

bulbil: small or immature bulb.

calyx: collective word for total number of sepals.

capsule: vessel containing seeds which when ripe usually splits open and expels the seeds at random.

carminative: a substance which relieves flatulence.

carpel: a division in the seed vessel.

clone: a product of vegetative propagation, being identical in all characteristics to that of the parent.

corolla: collective word for total number of petals.

cultivar: a variety or form taken from the wild and cultivated as a clone.

deciduous: a plant that loses its leaves in winter.

disc florets: small tubular florets typical . of the Compositeae family, forming tightly-packed yellow centre of flower (e.g. yarrow or daisy).

diuretic: a substance which stimulates the flow of urine.

drill: a shallow indentation or trench in which to sow seeds or lay rhizomes.

febrifuge: a medicinal substance to reduce fevers.

fibrous roots: many slender massed roots of fibrous nature (e.g. basil, chives).

florets: small individual flowers making up a head or cluster.

hastate: arrow-shaped.

'heel': the heel-shaped base of a cutting when a shoot is pulled downwards to detach it from a stem for propagation.

histamine: a substance present in the body which when released into the blood protects against infection from burns or wounds.

inflorescence: the arrangement or grouping of flowers on a plant.

island bed: a bed situated on a lawn or area to be viewed from all sides. It is best to put tall plants in the centre graduate heights down to low growing plants at the front edges.

internode: the space between nodes on a stem.

mucilage: a gummy, glutinous substance found in some plants, often soothing to inflamed areas of skin.

mulch: rotted leaves, lawn mowings, peat, compost and shredded bark used to spread over the ground around plants to give protection and help to conserve moisture in the soil. Mulch should not be spread on dry soil as it prevents the rain soaking down to the roots for some time.

node: the 'joint' on a stem from which leaf, flower or other stem buds develop.

pappus: fine hairy down which acts as a parachute for the dispersal of airborne seeds (e.g. dandelion and hemp agrimony).

pinnate: arrangement of leaflets in opposite pairs on common stalks.

radical leaves: those growing directly from the crown of the root (e.g. elecampane).

ray florets: small flowers having elongated or strap-shaped lobes, as the outer white florets of yarrow or daisy flowers.

rootstocks: gardener's term for the two or three year old mature roots which may be divided up, or from which growing buds can be cut, to form new young plants.

stipules: pairs of small, modified leaf-like structures at the base of the leaf stalk, giving protection to the bud.

'sport': a term used to describe a shoot or part of a plant which is out of character with the usual form and only by vegetative propagation can maintain its individual nature.

stolon: a horizontal stem at soil level which produces a new plant at its tip.

strobile: a cone shaped inflorescence made up of overlapping scales (e.g. hop).

styptic: an astringent substance used to arrest bleeding.

taproot: a thick, often tapering root, usually storing food (e.g. carrot, Hamburg parsley).

viable: capable of producing living growth; that is, germination of seeds.

vulnerary: a substance used in the treatment or healing of wounds.

INDEX

ENGLISH NAMES

Acanthus 20
Aconite 118
Agrimony 97
Alecost 28
Alkanet 20
Aloe 80
Angelica 10, 104
Anise 9, 11, 105

Balm 53; Golden variegated 53
Basil 52
Bay 16, 85
Bergamot 16, 54
Betony 54
Blue Caucasian Comfrey 24
Borage 21
Bugle 55
Burdock, Common 29; Greater 29

Calamint 56
Camphor plant 28
Caper Spurge 117
Caraway 106
Catmint 56
Catnip 57
Centaury 49
Chamomile 30
Chervil 107
Chickweed 26
Chicory 31
Chives 13, 81; Garlic 82
Clary 74
Clary Sage 75
Coltsfoot 31
Comfrey 10, 13; Blue Caucasian 24; Common 23; Red 25; Russian 24; Soft 25
Common Burdock 29
Common Mallow 87
Coriander 9, 107
Corn Salad 114
Cowslip 93
Creeping Thymes 79
Cumin 108
Curled Golden Marjoram 65
Curled Tansy 40
Curry Plant 32

Dandelion 32
Danewort 117
Deadly Nightshade 119
Dill 9, 108

Eau de Cologne Mint 68
Elder 27
Elecampane 13, 33
Evening Primrose 89
Eyebright 102

Fat Hen 47
Fennel 109
Feverfew 34; Golden 34
Figwort 102
Flax 9; Linseed 84; Perennial 84; red 84
Foxglove 118
French Tarragon 40

Garlic 81; Triangular-stalked 83
Garlic Chives 82
Garlic Mustard 43
Gipsywort 58
Goat's Rue 90
Golden Feverfew 34
Golden Lemon Thyme 79
Golden Marjoram 64
Golden Rod 35
Golden Thyme 79
Golden Tipped Marjoram 65
Golden Variegated Balm 53
Golden Variegated Sage 75
Good King Henry 46
Goosegrass 116
Great Mullein 103
Greater Burdock 29
Greater Plantain 92
Ground Ivy 58

Hemlock 121
Hemp Agrimony 35
Henbane 120
Herb Bennet 98
Hop 42
Horseradish 43
Horsetail 48
Houseleek 46
Hyssop 59

Lady's Mantle 98
Lady's Smock 44
Lavender 11, 16; Dutch or Grey Hedge 60; French 61; Hidcote Blue 61; Munstead 60; Old English 60; Pink 60; White 61
Lemon Thyme 78
Lemon Verbena 114
Liquorice 86
Linseed Flax 84
Loosestrife, Yellow 95
Lovage 13, 110
Lungwort 9, 22

Mace 37
Mallow, Common 87
Marigold 16, 36
Marjoram 13; Golden 64; Curled Golden 65; Golden Tipped 65; Pot 63
Marshmallow 89
Meadow Saffron 121
Meadowsweet 99
Melilot 86
Mignonette 96

Mint 9, 13, 16, 66; Apple 67; Apple Variegated 67; Bowles 67; Buddleia 67; Corsican 71; Eau de Cologne 68; Ginger 68; Lemon 68; Peppermint 70; Pennyroyal 71; Spearmint 69; Pineapple 68
Motherwort 72
Mugwort 9

Nasturtium 104
Nettle 112
Nightshade, Deadly 119

Orach 47
Oregano 62
Orris 51

Parsley 14, 16, 110
Pellitory of the Wall 113
Pennyroyal 71
Peppermint 70
Pilewort 95
Plantain, Greater 92; Rose 93
Pot Marjoram 63
Primrose 94
Purslane 93

Ramsons 82
Red Comfrey 25
Red Sage 75
Rocket 44; Sweet 44
Rosemary 11, 16, 72
Rose Plantain 92
Rue 9, 101
Russian Comfrey 24

Saffron 51; Meadow 121
Sage 16, 74; Clary 75; Golden Variegated 75; Red 75; Wood see Wood Sage
St John's Wort 50
Salad Burnet 97
Savory, Summer 76; Winter 13, 76
Scullcap 77
Self Heal 77
Silver Thyme 78
Sneezewort 37
Soapwort 27
Soft Comfrey 25
Solomon's Seal 91
Sorrel 90
Southernwood 38
Spearmint 69
Summer Savory 76
Sunflower 11, 39
Sweetbriar Rose 100
Sweet Cicely 111
Sweet Marjoram 62
Sweet Rocket 44

Tansy 40; Curled 40
Tarragon, French 40
Thornapple 120
Thyme 10, 13, 15, 16, 78;
  Creeping 79; Golden 79;
  Golden Lemon 79; Lemon
  78; Silver 78
Tree Onion 83
Triangular-stalked Garlic 83

Valerian 113
Verbena, Lemon 114
Vervain 115
Violet 114

Wild Strawberry 100
Wintergreen 48
Winter Savory 13, 76
Witch hazel 50
Woad 45
Woodruff 116
Wood Sage 80
Wormwood 38

Yarrow 41
Yellow Loosestrife 95

SCIENTIFIC NAMES

Acanthaceae 20
Acanthus mollis 20
Achillea decolorans 37;
  millefolium 41; *ptarmica*
  37
Aconitum napellus 118
Agrimonia eupatoria 96
Ajuga reptans 55
Alchemilla vulgaris 98
Alliaria petiolata 43
Allium cepa var. *proliferum*
  83; *moly* 83; *sativum* 81;
  schoenoprasum 81;
  triquetrum 83; *tuberosum*
  82; *ursinum* 82
Aloe Barbadensis 80; *vera*
  80
Aloysia triphylla 114
Althaea officinalis 89
Angelica Archangelica 104
Anethum graveolens 108
Anthemis nobilis 30
Anthriscus cerefolium 107
Arctium, lappa 29; *minus* 29
Armoracia rusticana 43
Artemisia abrotanum 38;
  absinthium 38;
  dracunculus 40
Asperula odorata 116
Atriplex hortensis 47
Atropa belladonna 119

Balsamita vulgaris 28
Betonica officinalis 54
Boraginaceae 20
Borago officinalis 21

Calamintha ascendens 56
Calendula officinalis 36
Cannabaceae 42
Caprifoliaceae 27, 117
Cardamine pratensis 44
Carum carvi 106
Caryophyllaceae 26
Chamaemelum nobile 30
Chenopodiaceae 46
Chenopodium album 47;
  Bonus Henricus 46
*Chrysanthemum balsamita
  tanacetoides* 28;
  parthenium 34;
  parthenium aureum 34
Cichorium intybus 31
Colchicum autumnale 121
Compositeae 28
Conium maculatum 121
Coriandrum sativum 107
Crassulaceae 46
Cruciferae 43
Crocus sativus 51
Cuminum cyminum 108

Datura stramonium 120
Digitalis purpurea 118

Equisetaceae 48
Equisetum arvense 48
Ericaceae 48
Eruca versicaria 44; *sativa*
  44
Erythraea centaurium 49
Eupatorium cannabinum 35
Euphorbiaceae 117
Euphorbia lathyrus 117
Euphrasia rostkoviana 102

Filipendula ulmaria 99
Foeniculum officinalis 109;
  vulgare 109
Fragaria vesca 100

Galega officinalis 90
Galium aparine 116
Gaultheria procumbens 48
Gentianaceae 49
Geum urbanum 98
Glechoma hederacea 58
Glycyrrhiza glabra 86
Guttiferae 50

Hamamelidaceae 50
Hamamelis virginiana 50
Helianthus annuus 39
Helichrysum angustifolium
  32; *plicatum* 32
Hesperis matronalis 44
Humulus lupulus 42
Hyoscyamus niger 120
Hypericum perforatum 50
Hyssopus officinalis 59

Inula Helenium 33
Iridaceae 51
Iris germanica var. *florentina*
  51
Isatis tinctoria 45

Labiateae 19, 52
Lavendula angustifolia 60;
  latifolia 60; *rosea* 60; *nana
  atropurpurea* 61; *nana
  alba* 61: *stoechas* 61
Lauraceae 85
Laurus nobilis 85
Leguminoseae 86, 90
Leonurus cardiaca 72
Levisticum officinale 110
Liliaceae 80, 121
Linaceae 84
Linum perenne 84;
  usitatissimum 84
Lippia citriodora 114
Lycopus europaeus 58
Lysimachia punctata 95

Malvaceae 87
Malva sylvestris 87
Melilotus officinalis 86
Melissa officinalis 53;
  officinalis variegata 53
Mentha 19; *aquatica cv.
  citrata* 68; *citrata cv.* 68;
  gentilis 68; *longifolia* 67; *x
  piperita* 19, 70; *x piperita
  cv. citrata* 68; *pulegium*
  71; *requienii* 71; *spicata*
  69; *suaveolens* 67;
  suaveolens rotundifolia
  var. *Bowles* 67;
  suaveolens variegata 67;
  viridis 69
Monarda didyma 54
Myrrhis odorata 111
Nepeta cataria 57; *faassenii*
  56; *mussini* 56

Ocimum basilicum 52
Oenothera biennis 89
Onagraceae 89
Origanum aureum 64;
  aureum crispum 65;
  marjorana 62; *onites* 63;
  vulgare 62; *vulgare
  variegatum* 65

Papilionaceae 90
Parietaria diffusa 113;
  officinalis 113
Pentaglottis sempervirens
  20
Petroselinum crispum 110
Phytolacca americana 90
Pimpinella anisum 105
Plantaginaceae 92
Plantago major 92; *major
  rosulatus* 93
Polygonaceae 90
Polygonatum multiflorum 91
Portulaca oleracea 93
Portulaceae 93
Poterium sanguisorba 97
Primulaceae 93
Primula veris 93; *vulgaris* 94
Prunella vulgaris 77
Pulmonaria officinalis 22

Ranunculaceae 95, 118
Ranunculus ficaria 95
Resedaceae 96
Reseda odorata 96
Rosaceae 96
Rosa rubiginosa 100
Rosmarinus officinalis 72
Rubiaceae 116
Rumex acetosa 90
Rutaceae 101
Ruta graveolens 101

Salvia horminum 74;
   officinalis 74; *officinalis
   icterina* 75; *officinalis
   purpurascens* 75; *sclarea*
   75
Sambucus ebulus 117; *nigra*
   27
Sanguisorba minor 97
Saponaria officinalis 27

Satureja hortensis 76;
   montana 76
Scrophulariceae 102, 118
Scrophularia nodosa 102
Scutellaria lateriflora 77
Sempervivum tectorum 46
Solanaceae 119
Solidago virgaurea 35
Stachys officinalis 54
Stellaria media 26
Symphytum Caucasicum 24;
   officinalis 23; *orientale* 25;
   rubrum 25; *x uplandicum*
   24

Tanacetum vulgare 40;
   vulgare crispum 40
Taraxacum officinale 32
Teucrium scorodonia 80
Thymus aureus 79;
   citriodorus 78; *citriodorus*

   aureus 79; *citriodorus*
   'Silver Queen' 78;
   serphyllum sps 79;
   vulgaris 78; *vulgaris*
   'Silver Posy' 78
Tropaeolaceae 104
Tropaeolum majus 104
Tussilago farfara 31

Umbellifereae 104, 121
Urticaceae 112
Urtica dioica 112

Valerianaceae 113
Valeriana officinalis 113
Valerianella locusta 114
Verbascum thapsus 103
Verbenaceae 114
Verbena officinalis 115
Violaceae 114
Viola odorata 114

ACKNOWLEDGEMENTS

The publishers wish to thank the following for their help in supplying
photographs for this book:

A-Z Collection 10, 94; Iris Hardwick Library 17; Nationalbibliothek
Osterreichische, Vienna 8.
All other photographs were kindly supplied by the author Madge Hooper.

The author and publishers would also like to acknowledge the kind help of
Dr J. R. Akeroyd of the Department of Botany, Reading University, in
advising on plant names and classification.